Managing the Menopause Without Oestrogen

Edited by

Margaret Rees and Tony Mander

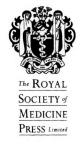

The ROYAL
SOCIETY *of*
MEDICINE
PRESS *Limited*

British Library Cataloguing in Publication Data

A catalogue record for this book is available from the British Library

ISBN 1 85315 592 6

Distribution in Europe and Rest of World:
Marston Book Services Ltd
PO Box 269
Abingdon
Oxon OX14 4YN, UK
Tel: +44 (0) 1235 465500
Fax: +44 (0) 1235 465555

Distribution in the USA and Canada:
Royal Society of Medicine Press Ltd
c/o Jamco Distribution Inc.
1401 Lakeway Drive
Lewisville TX 75057, USA
Tel: +1 800 538 1287
Fax: +1 972 353 1303
E-mail: jamco@majors.com

Distribution in Australia and New Zealand:
Elsevier Australia
30–52 Smidmore Street
Marrickville NSW 2204
Australia
Tel: + 61 2 9517 8999
Fax: + 61 2 9517 2249
E-mail: service@elsevier.com.au

Designed and Typeset by Phoenix Photosetting, Chatham, Kent

Printed in Great Britain by Marston Book Services Ltd , Oxford

List of contents

List of contributors

Paola Albertazzi
Senior Lecturer, Centre for Metabolic Bone, Hull Royal Infirmary, Hull, UK

Aedin Cassidy
Professor of Diet & Health, School of Medicine, Health Policy & Practice, University of East Anglia, Norwich, UK

Susan R Davis
Jean Hailes Professor of Women's Health, Department of Obstetrics and Gynaecology, Monash University, Clayton, Australia

Andrew Hextall
Consultant Obstetrician and Gynaecologist, St Albans City Hospital, St Albans, UK

Joy Hinson
Reader in Molecular and Cellular Endocrinology, Barts and the London, Queen Mary School of Medicine and Dentistry, London, UK

Alyson Huntley
Research Fellow, Complementary Medicine, Peninsula Medical School, Universities of Exeter and Plymouth, Exeter, UK

Clare E Kearney
Specialist Registrar in Obstetrics and Gynaecology, Women and Children's Hospital, Hull Royal Infirmary, Hull, UK

Brigid McKevith
Nutrition Scientist, British Nutrition Foundation, High Holborn House, London, UK

Alfred O Mueck

Head of the Department of Endocrinology and Menopause, Department of Obstetrics and Gynaecology, University of Tuebingen, Tuebingen, Germany

Martin K Oehler

Clinical Fellow, Department of Obstetrics and Gynaecology, Monash Medical Centre, Melbourne, Australia

Ulrika Pettersson

Clinical Lecturer in Rheumatology, Department of Medicine and Therapeutics, Medical School, Aberdeen, UK

Peter Raven

Senior Lecturer in Psychiatry, Metabolic and Clinical Trials Unit, Department of Mental Health Sciences, Royal Free and University College Medical School, University College London, London, UK

Margaret Rees

Reader in Reproductive Medicine, Nuffield Department of Obstetrics and Gynaecology, John Radcliffe Hospital, Oxford, UK

David M Reid

Professor of Rheumatology, Department of Medicine and Therapeutics, Medical School, Aberdeen, UK

Harald Seeger

Head of Endocrinology and Menopause Laboratory, Department of Obstetrics and Gynaecology, University of Tuebingen, Tuebingen, Germany

Andrew Sinclair

Specialist Registrar in Urology, Manchester Royal Infirmary, Manchester, UK

Dani Singer

Menopause Counsellor, Department of Obstetrics and Gynaecology, Menopause Clinic Research Unit, Northwick Park Hospital, Harrow, Middlesex, UK

Christopher Smejkal

Microbiology Research Fellow, School of Animal and Microbial Sciences, University of Reading, Reading, Berkshire, UK

Elizabeth A Thompson

Consultant Homeopathic Physician and Honorary Senior Lecturer in Palliative Medicine. Bristol Homeopathic Hospital, Bristol, UK

Joanna Thompson Coon
Research Fellow, Complementary Medicine, Peninsula Medical School, Universities of Exeter and Plymouth, Exeter, UK

Leila Hellevi Toiviainen
Philosophy Lecturer, School of Philosophy, University of Tasmania, Hobart, Tasmania *and* Department of Moral and Social Philosophy, University of Helsinki, Helsinki, Finland

Preface

Publication of the results of the combined and oestrogen-alone arms of the Women's Health Initiative and the Million Women Study has lead to increasing interest in the use of alternatives to hormone replacement therapy (HRT). Women and health professionals are concerned about the controversies surrounding breast cancer and cardiovascular disease risk in association with HRT.

Management of postmenopausal women is now a multidisciplinary public health issue as life expectancy is rising. Menopause management is no longer solely the remit of gynaecologists, but also involves other disciplines, such as general physicians, geriatricians, cardiologists and orthopaedic surgeons as well as general practitioners and nurse specialists. In the UK average female life expectancy is 81 years, which means that women can expect to live for 30 years after the menopause. Currently one-third of women are aged over 50. Increasing longevity results in altered interpersonal relationships and more reliance on women as carers for elderly relatives. This affects current social structures and the need for health service provision. Some conditions associated with older females, such as osteoporotic hip fracture, can lead to permanent disability and loss of independence. It is thus essential to develop a wide range of strategies that can be targeted to individual women and will help them to maintain good health, independence and quality of life throughout their postmenopausal years.

The aim of this book is to provide up-to-date evidence on the role and safety of non-oestrogen based strategies. Experts have written chapters covering many aspects of standard pharmacopoeia and surgical procedures, alternative and complementary therapies, and lifestyle interventions. The chapters are intentionally concise to create an easy to read, 'dip-in' book for the busy health professional dealing with postmenopausal women. The further reading lists, found at the end of each chapter, are a selection of relevant up-to-date publications.

Margaret Rees

Tony Mander

Pharmacological and surgical interventions

1

Statins

Alfred O Mueck and Harald Seeger

Introduction
Clinical benefits of statins

Rationale for a statin/hormone
    replacement therapy combination
Further reading

Introduction

The statins are probably the most interesting class of drugs to have been developed over the past 30 years. They exert their actions mainly by inhibiting the key enzyme of cholesterol biosynthesis HMG-CoA-reductase (3-hydroxy-3-methylglutaryl-coenzyme A) (Figure 1). This enables them to influence lipid metabolism –

an effect that was for a long while the exclusive focus of attention and the rationale for classifying the statins primarily as 'lipid-lowering drugs'. Statins are now increasingly being found to have direct vascular actions that improve endothelial function and to exert a variety of protective effects against the development and progression of atherosclerosis. This seems to have far-reaching clinical

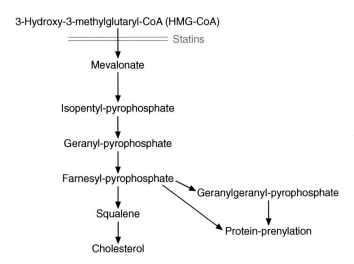

Figure 1
Cholesterol biosynthetic pathway.

significance, as the mechanisms behind the actions of the statins evidently take effect in the cardiovascular system much more rapidly than can be explained in terms of changes in lipid profiles. Most recently, mechanisms involving plaque stabilization or even direct antiarrhythmic actions have been postulated for statins in studies that evaluated their potential utility in the treatment of acute coronary syndrome.

Very recent findings that indicated that statins might also be valuable in the prevention and treatment of osteoporosis and dementia have come as a surprise. Particular interest also focuses on the newly discovered potency of statins in inhibiting the proliferation of certain malignancies, including breast cancer, at least in experimental *in vitro* models.

Clinical benefits of statins

Cardiovascular protection

Cardiovascular diseases head the list of causes of death in menopausal women, with a rate that is even higher than mortality from cancer. Statin therapy undoubtedly is effective in the primary and secondary prevention of cardiovascular diseases in both sexes. Reductions in mortality of up to 30% have been recorded in various studies – for premenopausal and postmenopausal women. More recently, a protective effect against cerebrovascular accident in patients with coronary heart disease has been the subject of debate. Interventional studies in this area, however, have only just started. Reportedly, beneficial endothelial effects (that is non-lipid effects) have been observed, although the effects of individual statins can differ considerably. Statins presumably also will be useful for effective primary prevention of coronary heart disease. At present, however, they are not recommended for postmenopausal women, especially in those with only mild hypercholesterolaemia, presumably mainly because of cost.

Osteoporosis prophylaxis

In 1999, a publication of a study in rodents surprisingly postulated for the first time that statins might have osteoprotective properties. The putative mechanism of action is that osteoblast stimulation is induced indirectly via osteoclast inhibition.

At least six analyses are available from data pools, and study reanalyses have been conducted to determine the extent to which statins can reduce osteoporosis-related risk of fracture. The data, however, are inconsistent. A recent prospective study did not indicate any benefit of statins on the risk of fracture and on bone density in postmenopausal women.

Alzheimer's disease

The close relation between disorders of cholesterol metabolism and Alzheimer's disease (for example, with respect to the role of cholesterol in the biosynthesis of β-amyloid) has been studied extensively. Recently, Alzheimer's patients have been shown to have raised concentrations of cholesterol in blood and cerebral tissue, as well as cholesterol levels that correlate with the extent of intracerebral β-amyloid deposits. It therefore came as no surprise that statins, as inhibitors of cholesterol biosynthesis, can also reduce β-amyloid secretion in neuronal cell lines – an effect also only known of late. This application for the statins needs to be examined in clinical trials.

Cancer

Occasional debate has considered whether statins induce malignancy. A recent meta-analysis of five randomized studies of not less than four years' duration involving at least 1000 patients and including a variety of statins and malignancies, however, showed that up to five years of statin therapy is not associated with an increased risk of cancer.

Initial *in vitro* studies showed that statins can prevent the growth of human breast cancer cells; oestrogen receptor-negative and -positive cells are influenced in a similar manner, although the effect is more pronounced in receptor-negative cells. A recent trial indicated that use of statins might lead to nearly 70% reductions in rates of breast cancer in older women; however, the data were based on a small number of breast cancer events.

Rationale for a statin/hormone replacement therapy combination

Clinical evidence of the value of combining hormone replacement therapy (HRT) and statins, especially for cardiovascular prevention, has been produced up to now only by the Heart and Estrogen/progestin Replacement Study (HERS). This study so far has been the only randomized, double-blind, placebo-controlled study on secondary prevention with clinical endpoints (such as myocardial infarction and mortality) to investigate a relatively high patient number for a study period of 4.1 years. Some women were treated with lipid-lowering agents, especially statins, in addition to HRT. At study inception, these patients accounted for 18% of the total sample of 1380 users of HRT; while in the placebo group the proportion was significantly higher (22%). Statins consequently were argued to confer a prognostic improvement in the placebo group. As the statistical adjustment for this difference did not produce any change in the overall result, this conclusion is somewhat open to question. During the study, 47% of the patients who took HRT and 45% of those who received placebo were treated with lipid-lowering drugs, especially statins, and one notable finding was a 50% reduced risk of thrombosis for those who took statins.

Lipid metabolism – proven additive effects

At present, the combination of statins and HRT is used almost exclusively to achieve an improvement in the lipid profile of symptomatic postmenopausal women with hypercholesterolaemia. Several studies have already shown that combining statins with oestrogen can provide an improvement, although this was not always significant for all lipid components. The two drug classes seem to exert differing effects on lipids.

These studies proved that statins as well as (oral) HRT can increase concentrations of high-density lipoprotein (HDL) cholesterol and reduce concentrations of low-density lipoprotein (LDL) cholesterol and that these effects almost always were significant. The benefit was usually enhanced by the combination, with statins exerting more potent effects on LDL cholesterol and (oral) oestrogen having a greater action on HDL cholesterol. Statins, however, also reduce concentrations of triglycerides, which often are raised by oral oestrogen replacement. Although the clinical relevance may be contentious, the changes observed will definitely be of practical significance in specific cases – for example in women with lipid disorders. Oestrogens, on the other hand, can reduce lipoprotein (a). Regarded as an independent risk factor for cardiovascular diseases, lipoprotein (a) is an important marker for the clotting/fibrinolytic process and for lipid metabolism. Statins, like almost all other lipid-lowering agents, have no effect on lipoprotein (a). The combination of hormones with statins is thus particularly beneficial in terms of these risk markers.

Vascular non-lipid effects

The possibility that statins may exert direct vascular effects has only recently stimulated interest. We have explored 'non-lipid effects' of oestrogens and statins and have seen beneficial effects of both on all markers, although the statins are more effective. In terms of markers of endothelial function, such as prostacyclin and endothelin (the most vasodilatory and vasoconstrictory endothelial mediators, respectively), the combination of the two

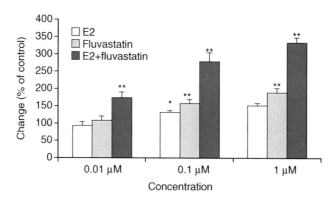

Figure 2
Changes in synthesis of endothelial prostacyclin in human umbilical veins after addition of fluvastatin and 17β-oestradiol (E2) alone and in equimolar combinations. Means ± SD from duplicates of three different experiments. *p value <0.05. **p value <0.01.

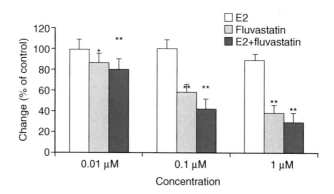

Figure 3
Changes in synthesis of endothelial endothelin in human umbilical veins after addition of fluvastatin (Flu) and 17β-oestradiol (E2) alone and in equimolar combinations. Values expressed as percentage of control value (100%). Means ± SD from duplicates of three different experiments. *p value <0.05. **p value <0.01.

substances produced an additive effect (Figures 2 and 3).

Choosing hormone replacement therapy/statin combinations

At present, the general tendency is to selectively combine HRT with a statin, with the aim of achieving a significant effect on the lipid profile – for example, in women with severe hypercholesterolaemia. The use of the two drug groups should be guided mainly by the known effects of each component. The increase in HDL cholesterol seen with conventional statins is not particularly large. This might be why the studies performed so far with a combination of statins and HRT were limited to the use of oral oestrogens, specifically equine oestrogens, with the aim of achieving a more powerful effect.

Adverse drug reactions and drug interactions should receive more attention, especially during long-term therapy of the elderly. This aspect can and should be a major cofactor when deciding in favour of a specific HRT/statin combination. The choice naturally also depends on the therapeutic indication, such as the initial lipid profile, which can also be influenced by the type of HRT. As for the 'non-lipid' effects, close attention also should be paid to the progestogen component. Indeed, differences in the direct vascular actions of progestogens have been shown, and these in turn can have a significant impact on endothelial function, the development and progression of atherosclerosis or factors such as plaque stability.

Further reading

Archer DF. Progestogen effects on coronary arteries: the need for definitive clinical trials. *Menopause* 2001; **8**: 1–2.

Bjerre LN, LeLorier J. Do statins cause cancer? A meta-analysis of large randomized clinical trials. *Am J Med* 2001; **110**: 738–40.

Cauley JA, Zmuda JM, Lui LY, *et al*. Lipid-lowering drug use and breast cancer in older women: a prospective study. *J Women's Health* 2003; **12**: 749–56.

Fak AS, Erenus M, Tezcan H, *et al* . Effects of simvastatin alone or in combination with continuous combined hormone replacement therapy on serum lipid levels in hypercholesterolaemic post-menopausal women. *Eur Heart J* 2000; **21**: 190–7.

Gaw A, Packard CJ, Shepherd J. *Statins: the HMG CoA reductase inhibitors in perspectives*. London: Martin Dunitz Publishing, 2000.

Grady E, Wenger NK, Herrington D, *et al*. Postmenopausal hormone therapy increases risk of venous thromboembolic disease. The Heart and Estrogen/progestin Replacement Study HERS). *Ann Intern Med* 2000; **132**: 689–96.

Hulley ST, Grady D, Bush T, *et al*. For the heart and estrogen/progestin replacement study (HERS) research group. Randomized trial of estrogen plus progestin for secondary prevention of coronary heart disease in postmenopausal women. *JAMA* 1998; **280**: 605–13.

LaCroix AZ, Cauley JA, Pettinger M, *et al*. Statin use, clinical fracture, and bone density in postmenopausal women: Results from the Women's Health Initiative Observational Study. *Ann Intern Med* 2003; **139**: 97–104.

Meier CR, Schlienger RG, Draenzlin ME, *et al*. HMG-CoA reductase inhibitors and risk of fractures. *JAMA* 2000; **283**: 3205–10.

Mueck AO, Seeger H. Statins and direct vascular actions. *Panminerva Medica* 2003; **45**: 1–6.

Mueck AO, Seeger H, Deuringer FU, Wallwiener D. Effect of estrogen/statin combination on biochemical markers of endothelial function in human coronary cell cultures. *Menopause* 2001; **8**: 216–21.

Mueck AO, Seeger H, Wallwiener D. Fluvastatin combined with 17ß-estradiol: effect on the oxidation of human low density lipoprotein. *Exp Clin Endocrinol Diabetes* 2000; **108**: 316–18.

Mundy G, Garrett R, Harris S, *et al*. Stimulation of bone formation *in vitro* and in rodents by statins. *Science* 1999; **286**: 1946–9.

Reid IR, Hague W, Emberson J, *et al*. Effect of pravastatin on frequency of fracture in the LIPID study; secondary analysis of a randomised controlled trial. *Lancet* 2001; **357**: 509–12.

Seeger H, Lippert C, Wallwiener D, Mueck AO. Estradiol effect combined with fluvastatin on the production of prostacyclin and endothelin in human umbilical vein endothelial cells. *Pharm Pharmacol Lett* 2000; **1**: 16–18.

Seeger H, Wallwiener D, Mueck AO. Statins can inhibit proliferation of human breast cancer cells *in vitro*. *Exp Clin Endocrinol Diabetes* 2003; **111**: 47–8.

Simons M, Keller P. Cholesterol depletion inhibits the generation of beta-amyloid in hippocampal neurons. *Proc Natl Acad Sci USA* 1998; **95**: 6460–4.

Van Staa TP, Wegman S, de Vries F, *et al*. Use of statins and risk of fractures. *JAMA* 2001; **285**: 1850–5.

2 Antiresorptive agents

Ulrika Pettersson and David M Reid

Introduction

In postmenopausal women, bone loss results from an increased rate of bone remodelling, with an imbalance between bone resorption and formation. Normally, approximately 10% of the bone surface undergoes remodelling at any one time. Bone turnover takes place in focal and discrete packets within the skeleton, and it progresses in a systematic fashion, with resorption undertaken by osteoclasts and followed by formation undertaken by osteoblasts – a phenomenon called coupling (Figure 1). If these two processes are not matched, an imbalance will occur that will result in irreversible bone loss. Postmenopausal bone loss occurs in two phases: a rapid phase, starting at around the menopause and lasting

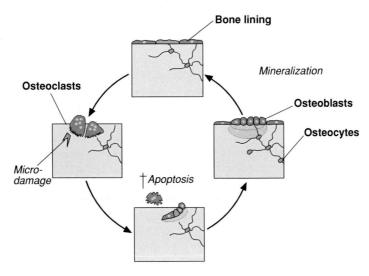

Figure 1
Bone turnover and the bone remodelling cycle. Adapted and reproduced with permission from Stuart H Ralston, University of Aberdeen.

Table 1
Antifracture efficacy of different interventions in postmenopausal osteoporotic women: grade of recommendations by the Royal College of Physicians.

Intervention	Spine	Non-vertebral	Hip
		Fracture	
Alendronate	A	A	A
Calcitonin	A	B	B
Calcitriol	A	A	ND
Calcium	A	B	B
Calcium + vitamin D	ND	A	A
Cyclic etidronate	A	B	B
Raloxifene	A	ND	ND
Risedronate	A	A	A
Tibolone	ND	ND	ND
Vitamin D	ND	B	B

Grading of evidence is classified as follows:
A = meta-analysis of randomized controlled trials (RCT) or from at least one RCT or at least one well designed controlled study without randomization.
B = from at least one other type of well designed quasi-experimental study or from designed non-experimental descriptive studies, eg comparative studies, correlation studies, case-control studies.
C = from expert committee reports/opinions and/or clinical experience of authorities.
ND = not detected.

for about five years (around 2–3% loss per year), followed by a slow, more generalized loss (about 0.5% loss per year). Oestrogen deficiency that causes increased osteoclast activity is the major mechanism that underlies the rapid phase, whereas parathyroid activity and impaired osteoblast function cause the slow, age-related phase.

All antiresorptive drugs act by inhibiting osteoclast activity, thus reducing the raised levels of bone turnover seen after menopause. The treatment alternatives discussed in this chapter include all antiresorptive compounds that are currently approved for treatment of postmenopausal osteoporosis in the UK, except hormone replacement therapy. The Royal College of Physicians' grading of efficacy of treatments is given in Table 1. An anabolic alternative recently became available for the treatment of severe osteoporosis: teriparatide is a recombinant DNA agent that consists of the first 34 amino acids of parathyroid hormone.

Calcium and vitamin D as adjunctive therapy

Adequate intake of calcium and vitamin D is necessary for prevention and treatment of osteoporosis. Although dietary calcium is as effective as pharmacological agents, supplements might be required when intake is low. Calcium is absorbed in the gut by active transport, which is facilitated by vitamin D. Serum levels of vitamin D normally decrease with age because of reduced intake, impaired synthesis in the skin and low exposure to sunshine. As the main source of vitamin D is endogenous production, seasonal variations result in lower concentrations during the winter. In countries in Northern latitudes, vitamin D deficiency is especially common in the elderly. The clinical impact of calcium and/or vitamin D supplementation has been investigated in several studies, with varying outcomes. A recent meta-analysis of 15 trials found that calcium supplementation alone had a small positive effect on bone density in the lumbar spine and hip. The study also found that calcium tended to lower the risk for vertebral fractures (relative risk 0.77 [95% confidence interval], 0.54–1.09), whereas a possible reduction of hip fractures was more uncertain (relative risk 0.86, 0.43–1.72). It should be noted that an antifracture benefit of calcium has not been found in perimenopausal women or in early postmenopausal women (<5 years after the menopause). Most studies suggest that a daily intake of 1000–1200 mg calcium is necessary to preserve bone health in postmenopausal women.

Vitamin D alone has also been tried as treatment for osteoporosis, but again with variable results. In a Finnish study in elderly women, annual injections of 150,000–300,000 IU vitamin D reduced the rate of all clinical fractures, whereas other studies have shown no effect on fracture incidence of vitamin D in daily doses of 300–400 IU. Several prospective studies of combined calcium and vitamin D supplementation have, however, shown positive results. Daily supplementation with 500–1200 mg calcium in combination with 700–800 IU vitamin D was thus associated with a significantly lower rate of hip fractures in institutionalized as well as healthy independently living women compared with placebo, which suggests that supplementation with calcium plus vitamin D is associated with a better benefit than either nutrient alone. A recent study also showed that calcium and vitamin D replacement reduced body sway and falls in elderly people with deficiencies of the two substances – probably by improving muscle power and balance.

Antiresorptive drugs

Antiresportive drugs include bisphosphonates, selective oestrogen receptor modulators (SERMs), calcitonin and calcitriol.

Bisphosphonates

Bisphosphonates are synthetic pyrophosphate analogues that bind to hydroxyapatite in bone and inhibit resorption by decreasing the number and activity of osteoclasts. On the basis of their structure and mechanism of action, they can be classified into two groups:

- non-nitrogen containing bisphosphonates, such as etidronate, which are of low potency and inhibit osteoclast function via metabolism into toxic adenosine triphosphate metabolites that cause cell death
- nitrogen containing bisphosphonates, such as alendronate and risedronate, which inhibit farnesyl pyrophosphate synthase (FPPS), an enzyme of the mevalonate pathway. This results in inhibition of the prenylation of small guanosine triphosphate binding proteins in osteoclasts, which leads to reduced resorptive activity and accelerated cell death.

Three bisphosphonates are currently approved in the UK for postmenopausal osteoporosis: etidronate, alendronate and risedronate. All are poorly absorbed from the gut and must be taken on an empty stomach. Typically, only 1–3% of the given dose is absorbed. The most common side-effect of bisphosphonates is gastrointestinal discomfort; however, it is less common with the new weekly regimens. Bisphosphonates are currently the best studied agents for prevention of bone loss and reduction in fractures, and they are the only ones approved for reduction of hip fracture. Optimal duration of treatment is unknown, and some concerns have been raised about the risk of 'frozen bone': that long-term treatment with potent bisphosphonates might turn off remodelling completely, leading to augmented mineralization and accumulation of microdamage. Data are awaited.

Etidronate

Etidronate, which was the first bisphosphonate to be developed, is given as an intermittent cyclical therapy of 400 mg daily for 14 days followed by 500 mg calcium for 76 days. The first randomized, placebo-controlled trials with cyclical etidronate showed an increase in bone mineral density (BMD) of the spine by about 4% and a significant reduction of vertebral fracture rate after two years' treatment. This was later supported by a meta-analysis of 13 trials that found that etidronate lowered the risk of vertebral fractures with a relative risk of 0.63 (0.44–0.92). No effect was noted, however, for non-vertebral fractures. In a post-marketing retrospective cohort study with a general practice research database including 7977 patients on cyclical etidronate therapy, however, the risk of non-vertebral fracture was reduced by 20% and of hip fracture by 34% relative to age- and sex-matched control patients with osteoporosis. Etidronate is generally well tolerated and does not seem to cause any gastrointestinal symptoms.

Alendronate

Alendronate, an aminobisphosphonate, is a second generation bisphosphonate and a potent inhibitor of bone turnover. Multiple long-term studies have showed that it maintains and increases BMD of the hip and spine in postmenopausal women. Changes are most marked in the first year but BMD continues to increase up to at least 10 years of treatment and seems to be maintained for at least two years after the drug is stopped. Alendronate reduces the incidence of vertebral and non-vertebral fractures by approximately 50% over 3–4 years in postmenopausal women with established osteoporosis. The risk of vertebral fractures is reduced in the first year of treatment. The approved dose for prevention of osteoporosis is 5 mg daily or 35 mg once weekly and for treatment of established disease is 10 mg daily or 70 mg once weekly. Weekly administration has the same efficacy as the daily dose regimen.

Risedronate

Risedronate, a pyridinyl bisphosphonate with potent antiresorptive activity, maintains and increases BMD of the hip and spine by 3–6% in postmenopausal women. At a dose of 5 mg daily, it reduces the cumulative incidence of new vertebral fractures by 41–49% over three years and 50% over five years in postmenopausal women with prevalent vertebral fractures. A significant effect is seen after six months of treatment. Recently the effect of risedronate on the incidence of hip fracture was assessed in a large study of postmenopausal women age >70 years. Three years' treatment produced a significant 30% overall reduction in hip fractures and a 40% reduction in a subset of women with established osteoporosis. No benefit was seen in a subgroup of women aged over 80 years with only non-skeletal risk factors for osteoporosis. The antifracture effect of risedronate was recently shown to continue after at least seven years of treatment. The approved dose for prevention and treatment of established disease is 5 mg daily or 35 mg once weekly; both regimens have similar efficacy.

Selective oestrogen receptor modulators (SERMs)

Selective estrogen receptor modulators are compounds that bind with a high affinity to oestrogen receptors and act as oestrogen agonists or antagonists depending on the target tissue (see Chapter 3). Raloxifene was the first SERM to be approved for prevention and treatment of postmenopausal osteoporosis. It acts as an oestrogen agonist in bone but an antagonist in breast and uterine tissues. In early postmenopausal women, a daily dose of 60 mg raloxifene prevented bone loss at all skeletal sites, with a 2–3% increase in BMD of the hip and spine compared with placebo. In a large randomized, placebo-controlled trial involving 7705 women with osteoporosis, treatment with 60 mg raloxifene (with daily supplements of 500 mg calcium and 400–600 IU vitamin D) was associated with 30% and 50%

reductions of the incidence of vertebral fractures in women with and without prevalent vertebral fractures, respectively. No effect was noted, however, in the rate of non-vertebral fractures.

Calcitonin

Calcitonin, a peptide secreted by the C cells in the thyroid gland, reduces bone loss by inhibiting osteoclasts. It can be given parenterally or as a nasal spray, the latter form being more favourable, as the former is associated with a high incidence of nausea, vomiting and facial flushing. Calcitonin produces small increments in bone mass of the spine in late postmenopausal women (>5 years after menopause), whereas no effect has been seen in cortical bone such as in the hip and forearm. Two randomized studies that evaluated the effects of nasal calcitonin on fracture risk both showed significant reductions in vertebral fractures. In the largest study, which involved 1255 postmenopausal women with established osteoporosis, intranasal calcitonin (200 IU/day) seemed to reduce the rate of vertebral fractures by about 33% relative to placebo, whereas no effect was found on hip fractures. The study was underpowered, however, and the high discontinuation rate excluded meaningful analysis of non-vertebral fractures. A recent meta-analysis also suggested that the benefits of calcitonin might be lower than those observed in studies on bisphosphonates. Calcitonin, however, also may have an analgesic benefit in patients with acute painful vertebral fractures. Treatment with calcitonin should therefore be considered for older women with osteoporosis with painful vertebral fractures and for those who fail to respond to or are intolerant of biphosphonates. Calcitonin should always be accompanied by optimal calcium and vitamin D intake.

Calcitriol

Calcitriol is a vitamin D analogue that facilitates the intestinal absorption of calcium and also exerts a direct effect on bone cells. Clinical trials that assessed the effect of calcitriol on bone have produced conflicting results, mainly because of small sample sizes. In the largest study (622 osteoporotic women), which was not placebo-controlled or double blind, the rate of new vertebral fractures was significantly lower in women treated with calcitriol compared with those women who received calcium alone. A decrease in non-vertebral fractures was also seen in the calcitriol group. The result, however, might have been biased by an unusually high increase of the annual fracture rate in the calcium group. The potential dangers of hypercalcaemia and hypercalciuria from high doses of calcitriol means that serum and urine calcium concentrations should be monitored closely.

Anabolic therapies

Parathyroid hormone

Parathyroid hormone (PTH), especially intact human PTH [hPTH(1-84)] and various fragments [particularly hPTH(1–34)], have been investigated for the treatment of osteoporosis. Teriparatide, the 1–34 genetically engineered fragment, was licensed for prescription in 2003 to be used in a dose of 20 µg given by daily subcutaneous injection for 18 months. Its anabolic action stimulates osteoblasts to a greater extent than osteoclasts.

The pivotal randomized controlled trial was undertaken in 1637 postmenopausal women with prior vertebral fractures randomized to receive 20 or 40 µg PTH (1–34) or placebo. New vertebral fractures occurred in 14% of women who received placebo and 5% and 4%, respectively, of women who received 20 µg and 40 µg PTH. The respective relative risks of fracture in the women who received 20 µg and 40 µg PTH compared with those who received placebo were 0.35 (0.22–0.55) and 0.31 (0.19–0.50), respectively. New non-vertebral fragility fractures occurred in 6% of women in the placebo group and 3% of those in each PTH group [relative risks 0.47 (0.25–0.88) and 0.46 (0.25–0.861), respectively]. No significant reduction in hip fracture was found. The 40 µg dose increased BMD at the lumbar spine more than the 20 µg dose, but it had similar effects on the risk of fracture and was more likely to have side-effects, hence the chosen marketed dose of 20 µg daily. When combined with alendronate no synergy in effect has been found and so the two should not be co-prescribed.

Future developments

Another interesting option in development is strontium ranelate. Strontium can participate in bone mineralization in place of calcium, and, although the cellular mechanisms still are being investigated, evidence suggests effects on osteoclasts and osteoblasts. Unlike the effect of antiresorptive agents, with which a reduction in resorption is followed by a coupled reduction in formation, the studies of strontium indicate a tendency to reduce bone resorption while bone formation remains stable or is increased. Conservation of bone mass and reduction in fractures have been reported.

Conclusion

Prevention and treatment of osteoporosis should be based on an assessment of the patient's risk of fracture and on the efficacy and adverse effects of the drugs likely to be prescribed.

Although raloxifene and calcitonin only seem to reduce the risk of vertebral fractures, alendronate and risedronate are associated with a reduction of fractures at all sites and therefore provide the most potent clinical benefit of the currently available antiresorptive drugs. The impact of teriparatide needs to be ascertained. An adequate intake of calcium and vitamin D is an important component in all types of treatment for osteoporosis and for the very elderly, frail and housebound patients,

supplementation with vitamin D and calcium alone might be enough to reduce the risk of hip fractures.

Further reading

Barrett-Connor E, Grady D, Sashegyi A, et al. Raloxifene and cardiovascular events in osteoporotic postmenopausal women: Four-year results from the MORE (Multiple Outcomes of Raloxifene Evaluation) randomized trial. JAMA 2002; **287**: 847–57.

Black DM, Cummings SR, Karpf DB, et al. Randomised trial of effect of alendronate on risk of fracture in women with existing vertebral fractures. Lancet 1996; **348**: 1535–41.

Black DM, Greenspan SL, Ensrud KE et al. The effects of parathyroid hormone and alendronate alone or in combination in postmenopausal osteoporosis. N Engl J Med 2003; **349**: 1207–15.

Bone HG, Hosking D, Devogelaer J-P, et al. Ten years' experience with Alendronate for osteoporosis in postmenopausal women. N Engl J Med 2004; **350**: 1189–99.

Cauley JA, Norton L, Lippman ME, et al. Continued breast cancer risk reduction in postmenopausal women treated with raloxifene: 4-year results from the MORE trial. Breast Cancer Res Treat 2001; **65**: 125–34.

Chapuy MC, Arlot ME, Duboeuf F, et al. Vitamin D3 and calcium to prevent hip fractures in elderly women. N Engl J Med 1992; **327**: 1637–42.

Chesnut III CH, Silverman S, Andriano K, et al. A randomized trial of nasal spray salmon calcitonin in postmenopausal women with established osteoporosis: the prevent recurrence of osteoporotic fractures study. Am J Med 2000; **109**: 267–76.

Cranney A, Guyatt G, Krolicki B, et al. A meta-analysis of etidronate for the treatment of postmenopausal osteoporosis. Osteoporosis Int 2001; **12**: 140–51.

Dawson-Hughes B, Harris SS, Krall EA, et al. Effect of calcium and vitamin D supplementation on bone density in men and women 65 years of age or older. N Engl J Med 1997; **337**: 670–6.

Emkey R, Reid I, Mulloy A, et al. Ten-year efficacy and safety of alendronate in the treatment of osteoporosis in postmenopausal women. J Bone Miner Res 2002; **17**: S319.

Harris ST, Watts NB, Genant HK, et al. Effects of risedronate treatment on vertebral and nonvertebral fractures in women with postmenopausal osteoporosis. JAMA 1999; **282**: 1344–52.

Heikenheimo RK, Inkovaara JA, Harju EJ, et al. Annual injection of vitamin D and fractures of aged bone. Calcif Tissue Int 1992; **51**: 105–10.

Lips P, Graafmans WC, Ooms ME, et al. Vitamin D supplementation and fracture incidence in elderly persons: a randomized, placebo-controlled clinical trial. Ann Intern Med 1996; **124**: 400–6.

Lyritis GP, Tsakalakos N, Magiasis B, *et al*. Analgesic effect of salmon calcitonin in osteoporotic vertebral fractures: a double blind placebo-controlled study. *Calcif Tissue Int* 1991; **49**: 369–72.

McClung MR, Geusens P, Miller MD, *et al*. Effect of risedronate on the risk of hip fracture in elderly women. *N Engl J Med* 2001; **344**: 333–40.

Meunier PJ, Roux C, Seeman E, *et al*. The effects of strontium ranelate on the risk of vertebral fracture in women with postmenopausal osteoporosis. *N Engl J Med* 2004; **350**: 459–68.

Neer RM, Arnaud CD, Zanchetta JR, *et al*. Effect of parathyroid hormone (1–34) on fractures and bone mineral density in postmenopausal women with osteoporosis. *N Engl J Med* 2001; **344**: 1434–41.

Royal College of Physicians. *Osteoporosis: clinical guidelines for prevention and treatment. London, Royal College of Physicians. Update on pharmacological interventions and an algorithm for management.* London: Royal College of Physicians, 2001.

Schnitzer T, Bone HG, Crepaldi G, *et al*. Alendronate 70 mg once weekly is therapeutically equivalent to alendronate 10 mg daily for the treatment of postmenopausal osteoporosis. *Aging Clin Exp Res* 2000; **12**: 1–12.

Shea B, Wells G, Cranney A, *et al*. Meta-analysis of calcium supplementation for the prevention of postmenopausal osteoporosis. *Endocr Rev* 2002; **23**: 552–9.

Sorensen OH, Crawford GM, Mulder H, *et al*. Long-term efficacy of risedronate: a 5-year placebo-controlled clinical experience. *Bone* 2003; **32**: 120–6.

Tilyard MW, Spears GF, Thomson J, Dovey S. Treatment of postmenopausal osteoporosis with calcitriol or calcium. *N Engl J Med* 1992; **326**: 357–62.

3 Selective oestrogen receptor modulators (SERMs)

Clare E Kearney

Introduction
What is a SERM?
Tamoxifen

Raloxifene
New developments
Further reading

Introduction

The increasing loss of public confidence in the use of conventional oestrogen therapy means that the search for an alternative takes on a new significance. *In vivo* manipulation of oestrogen action is important not only in the management of menopausal symptoms and oestrogen dependent tumours but also in a variety of conditions in which oestrogen seems to have a role.

What is a SERM?

Selective oestrogen receptor modulators (SERMs) comprise a range of compounds: triphenylethylenes, benzothiophenes, benzopyrans, tetrahydronaphthylenes and unique compounds such as levormeloxifene (Table 1). They interact with oestrogen receptors, cause conformational change and result in transcriptional activity in some tissues but not others. They display mixed oestrogen agonist/antagonist activity. Four SERMs currently are licensed for use: tamoxifen,

toremifene, raloxifene and clomiphene (Figure 1).

In the absence of a ligand, the oestrogen receptor lies quiescent within the cell nucleus and is surrounded by inhibitory heat shock proteins. Ligand binding frees the proteins and dimerization ensues. There are two types of oestrogen receptor – alpha oestrogen receptor (ERα) and beta oestrogen receptors (ERβ), which are located at different sites (Table 2). Alpha oestrogen receptors seem to be needed for most of the known oestrogenic responses, and differential activation of ERα and ERβ does not necessarily explain tissue selectivity.

Activation of either receptor can be affected by the degree of involvement of the two ligand-binding domains AF (activation function) 1 and 2, which in turn results in interaction with the appropriate DNA response element. Cells differ in their requirement to have both AF1 and AF2 activated to induce agonist activity, and this may explain tissue selectivity. Final gene

Table 1 Classes of SERM.			
Benzothiophene	Triphenylethylenes	Benzopyran	Other
• Raloxifene	• Clomiphene • Toremifene • Tamoxifen	• Ormeloxifene • CHF 4056	• Levormeloxifene

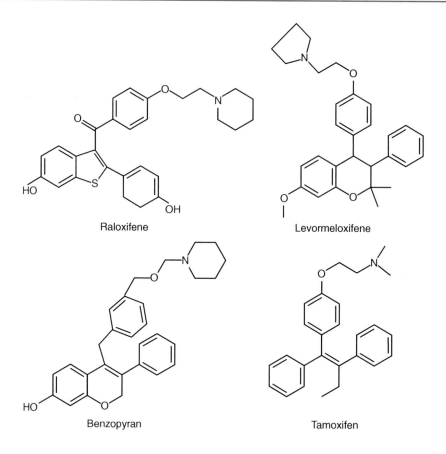

Figure 1
Structure of different SERMs.

Table 2
Distribution of α and β oestrogen receptors in the body.

System	α	β
Central nervous system	+	+
Ovary	+	+
Blood vessels	–	+
Bone	–	+
Lungs	–	+
Urogenital tract	–	+
Breast	+	–
Liver	+	–
Uterus	+	–

transcription can be altered further by recruitment of different coactivators and inhibitors, which also may be involved in tissue selectivity. For example, although tamoxifen and raloxifene are both oestrogenic in bone, only the former stimulates the endometrium.

Interest in the development of SERMs was stimulated in the 1950s with MER25, a triphenylethylene. In the 1970s, research into the antioestrogen clomiphene, a treatment for anovulation, and tamoxifen, a failed contraceptive being tested for the treatment of breast cancer, yielded interesting results.

Tamoxifen

In 1987, Jordon *et al* published the remarkable finding that rather than inducing osteoporosis the potent antioestrogen tamoxifen and the newly discovered keoxifene (raloxifene) maintained bone density in rats. Five years later, this finding was corroborated in a clinical study that showed a 0.61% increase per year in bone mineral density (BMD) of the lumbar spine.

Prolonged use of tamoxifen as adjuvant therapy in breast cancer resulted in investigation of its effects on the cardiovascular system. Tamoxifen has been shown to decrease the incidence of myocardial infarction and is thought to confer cardiovascular benefit by altering lipid and coagulation profiles (Table 3).

Table 3
The effect of tamoxifen on cardiovascular risk factors.

Cardiovascular risk factor	Change
Total cholesterol	decrease
LDL cholesterol	decrease
Apolipoprotein A	increase
Apolipoprotein B	decrease
Fibrinogen	decrease
Platelets	decrease

The difficulties inherent in receptor modulator research became apparent in 1985, when use of tamoxifen was linked with an increased risk of endometrial carcinoma. This risk was later quantified by the National Surgical Adjuvant Breast and Bowel Project as two in 1000 women.

Raloxifene

Raloxifene currently is the only SERM licensed for the treatment and prevention of postmenopausal osteoporosis. Interest at first was related to its *in vitro* ability to inhibit oestrogen dependent MCF7 breast cancer cells. Phase II clinical trials, however, failed to show that raloxifene was beneficial as a breast cancer treatment. Development of raloxifene was driven by its ability to maintain BMD in conjunction with favourable effects on cardiovascular risk factors.

Most data on raloxifene resulted from the Multiple Outcomes of Raloxifene Evaluation (MORE) study of over 7000 women with osteoporosis who were randomized to placebo, 60 mg/day raloxifene or 120 mg/day raloxifene. The licensed therapeutic dose is 60 mg/day.

Bone

After three years of treatment, patients who took raloxifene were found to have a significantly reduced risk of vertebral fracture (relative risk 0.7 [95% confidence interval 0.5–0.8]) but not hip fracture. This was true in women who had and had not had previous fractures. In women most at risk of subsequent fracture (those with severe vertebral fractures at the beginning of the trial), raloxifene reduced new vertebral fractures (relative risk 0.74 [0.54–0.99]; *p* value = 0.048) and non-vertebral fractures (clavicle, humerus, wrist, pelvis, hip and leg) (relative risk 0.53 [0.29–0.99]; *p* value = 0.046).

Increases in BMD with raloxifene were modest: 2.1% at the femoral neck and 2.6% at the spine. Analysis of bone tissue shows suppression of resorption and formation. This action is similar to that of other antiresorptive therapies, including oestrogen. It has been postulated that preservation of the microarchitecture of cancellous bone can be achieved without large increases in BMD. This may explain the apparently disproportionate decrease in fractures. Another possible explanation is that normalization of high bone turnover also plays an important role.

Cardiovascular effects of raloxifene

Studies of raloxifene have consistently shown reductions in concentrations of total cholesterol and LDL cholesterol. Concentrations of HDL cholesterol and triglycerides do not change significantly. In light of the results of the Heart and Estrogen/Progestin Replacement Study/Women's Health Initiative trial, it is evident that these essentially oestrogenic effects may not confer benefit.

As a result, 1035 women deemed to be at increased risk of cardiovascular disease in the Multiple Outcomes of Raloxifene Evaluation (MORE) study were reviewed. It should be remembered that the osteoporotic women in MORE were at low risk of cardiovascular events. Women who took raloxifene had a significantly lower risk of cardiovascular events (relative risk 0.6 [0.38–0.95]). No evidence showed that the first year of treatment was associated with an increased risk of cardiovascular events.

Raloxifene differs from oestrogen, in that it does not increase C-reactive protein or matrix metalloproteinase 9. Further work on a proinflammatory cause for cardiovascular disease therefore may be important. Together with the knowledge that apolipoprotein B, homocysteine and fibrinogen levels are lowered with raloxifene and that *in vitro* raloxifene seems to be a powerful antioxidant, hopes that raloxifene may be cardioprotective are high. The Raloxifene Use for the Heart (RUTH) study, which has completed recruitment (>10,000 women) and is due for publication in 2005, has been designed to resolve this issue.

Breast

Raloxifene decreased the risk of oestrogen receptor-positive breast cancers in the treatment arm of MORE by 84% (relative risk 0.16 [0.09–0.3]). The overall reduction in invasive breast cancer was 72% (relative risk 0.28 [0.17–0.46]). Raloxifene had no effect on oestrogen receptor-negative tumours. Further trials have been designed to examine this issue. Study of Tamoxifen and Raloxifene (STAR) is currently recruiting 22,000 women to evaluate the incidence of invasive breast cancer in high-

risk women. The RUTH study will also provide data about the risk of breast cancer.

Raloxifene does not increase breast pain and no increase in breast density (a risk factor for breast cancer), as determined by X-ray mammography, is noted.

Raloxifene and the uterus

Endometrial thickness was not increased in women who took raloxifene for five years. Treated women were no more likely to experience vaginal bleeding than those who took placebo. Although increased fluid in the endometrial cavity was found in one in 12 women on ultrasound examination, no endometrial abnormality was detected. The incidence of endometrial cancer of 0.77 per 1000 women years was the same in the placebo and treatment (60 mg) groups. The STAR study will determine whether raloxifene reduces the risk of endometrial cancer. Interestingly, development of levormeloxifene and idoxifene as treatments for osteoporosis was discontinued because of endometrial stimulation.

In animal studies (guinea pigs) as well as in women raloxifene shrank fibroids. This property may prove useful in the future.

In trials of levormeloxifene and idoxifene, women who took the treatment were more likely to undergo surgery for genitourinary prolapse than those who did not. Initial review of several raloxifene studies in which prolapse was not a primary outcome failed to show an increase in prolapse surgery. One small study with stringent analysis of prolapse suggests, however, that it may indeed be a complication of raloxifene therapy.

Risks

The most serious consequence of raloxifene therapy is a three-fold increase in the risk of venous thromboembolic disease, in line with tamoxifen and oestrogen therapy. The risk of deep venous thrombosis is seven per 1000 (raloxifene) versus two per 1000 (placebo), and the risks of pulmonary embolism are quoted as three per 1000 and one per 1000, respectively.

Minor side-effects include hot flushes, leg cramps and peripheral oedema: 24% of women who took raloxifene in the MORE study reported hot flushes. Most resolved within six months and discontinuation rates were less than 2%. No detrimental effect on cognitive function has been shown with raloxifene.

New developments

Many SERMs are being developed, primarily with the aim of preventing and treating postmenopausal osteoporosis

Arzoxifene, a third generation SERM, is undergoing Phase II clinical trials in the treatment of breast cancer and osteoporosis. It is thought that it may prove more effective than raloxifene. Phase III osteoporosis trials are planned to look at BMD, fracture risk reduction and incidence of invasive breast cancer.

Lasfoxifene, a bone protective agent, is the subject of the PEARL Phase III study of 7500 women.

Ospemifene is another SERM in the early stages of development in Scandinavia.

The problem of hot flushes remains with the newer SERMs and precludes their use in symptomatic, newly menopausal woman. In an attempt to counteract this problem, bazedoxifene is being trialled in the USA in conjunction with oestrogen therapy.

Further reading

Barrett-Conner E, Grady D, Sashegyi A, *et al.* Raloxifene and cardiovascular events in osteoporotic post menopausal women. *JAMA* 2002; **287**: 847–57.

Brzozokwsi am, Pike AC, Dauter Z, *et al.* Molecular basis of agonism and antagonism in the estrogen receptor. *Nature* 1997; **389**: 753–8.

Cauley JA, Norton L, Lippman ME, *et al.* Continued breast cancer risk reduction in postmenopausal women treated with raloxifene: 4-year results from the MORE trial. *Breast Cancer Research Treatment* 2001; **65**: 125–32.

Delmas PD, Genant HK, Crans GG, *et al.* Severity of prevalent vertebral fractures and the risk of subsequent vertebral and nonvertebral fractures: results from the MORE trial. *Bone* 2003; **33**: 522–32.

Ettinger B, Black DM, Mitlak BH, *et al.* Reduction of vertebral fracture risk in postmenopausal women with osteoporosis treated with raloxifene. *JAMA* 1999; **282**: 637–45.

Fischer B, Costantino JP, Redmond CK, *et al.* Endometrial cancer in tamoxifen treated breast cancer patients: findings NSABP B-14. *J Natl Cancer Inst* 1994; **86**: 527–37.

Goldstein SR, Neven P, Zhou L, *et al.* Raloxifene effect on frequency of surgery for pelvic floor relaxation. *Obstet Gynecol* 2001; **98**: 91–6.

Jireck S, Lee A, Pavo I, *et al.* Raloxifene prevents the growth of uterine leiomyomas in premenopausal women. *Fertil Steril* 2004; **81**: 132–6.

Jolly E, Bjarnason NH, Neven P, *et al.* Prevention of osteoporosis and uterine effects in postmenopausal women taking raloxifene for 5 years. *Menopause* 2003; **10**: 337–44.

Jordan VC, Phelps E, Lindgren JU. Effects of anti-estrogens on bone in castrated and intact female rats. *Breast Cancer Res Treat* 1987; **10**: 31–5.

Love RR, Mazess RB, Barden HS, *et al.* Effects of tamoxifen on bone mineral density in postmenopausal women with breast cancer. *N Engl J Med* 1992; **326**: 852–6.

Love RR, Weibe DA, Newcombe PA, *et al.* Effects of tamoxifen on cardiovascular risk factors in postmenopausal women. *Ann Int Med* 1991; **115**: 860–4.

McDonald C, Stewart HJ. Fatal myocardial infarction in the Scottish adjuvant tamoxifen trial. *BMJ* 1991; **303**: 435–7.

McDonnell DP, Chang CY, Norris JD, *et al.* Capitalizing on the complexities of estrogen receptor pharmacology in the quest for the perfect SERM. *Ann N Y Acad Sci* 2001; **949**: 16–35.

Nickelsen T, Lufkin EG, Riggs BL, *et al.* Raloxifene hydrochloride, a selective estrogen receptor modulator: safety assessment of effects on cognitive function and mood in postmenopausal women. *Psychoneuroendocriology* 1999; **24**: 115–28.

Porter KB, Tsibris JCM, Porter GW, *et al.* Effects of raloxifene in a guinea pig model for leiomyomas. *Am J Obstet Gynecol* 1998; **179**: 1283–7.

Riggs BL, Melton LJ. Bone turnover matters: the raloxifene treatment paradox of dramatic decreases in vertebral fractures without commensurate increases in bone density. *J Bone Min Research* 2002; **17**: 11–14.

Vardy MB, Lindsay R, Scotti RJ, *et al*. Short-term urogenital effects of raloxifene, tamoxifen, and estrogen. *Am J Obstet Gynecol* 2003; **189**: 81–8.

Varosy PD, Shlipak MG, Vittinghoff E, *et al*. Heart and Estrogen/Progestin Replacement Study (HERS) Investigators. Fracture and the risk of coronary events in women with heart disease. *Am J Med* 2003; **115**: 196–202.

Neurotransmitter modulation to treat hot flushes

Paola Albertazzi

Introduction

Hot flushes are associated so closely with the menopause as to be practically considered its hallmark. Although hot flushes are commonly thought to occur because of oestrogen withdrawal, other mechanisms may be involved. Many postmenopausal women do not suffer from hot flushes at all despite low endogenous oestrogen, and serum oestrogen levels are not correlated with the presence of hot flushes or with their intensity. Hot flushes, in fact, can be present in 15–25% of regularly menstruating women despite normal oestrogen levels and in postmenopausal women despite more than adequate doses of hormonal replacement therapy (HRT). Thus, although a fall in oestrogen concentration could be the first change, it might not directly be the cause of this symptom.

Despite the prevalence and bothersome nature of hot flushes, few studies have addressed their pathophysiology, and very little is known about the underlying mechanisms.

Neurotransmitter dysfunction in hot flushes

Hot flushes are a sudden sensation of heat or burning that starts in the head and neck area and then passes, often in waves, over the entire body but is particularly marked in the head, neck, upper chest and back. Hot flushes are a systemic symptom and are likely to arise from alterations in the central nervous system thermoregulatory set-point located in the anterior portion of the hypothalamus. Changes in body temperature are recognized by the thermoregulatory set-point centre that controls physiological responses that conserve or dissipate heat, such as vasodilatation or vasoconstriction of the skin. Indeed, the threshold between sweating and shivering – the interthreshold or neutral zone – is wide in premenopausal women, but it is much narrowed in postmenopausal women who suffer from hot flushes. Small changes in ambient temperature normally would not produce any major adaptive response, but in postmenopausal women with a low interthreshold zone, they may trigger major compensatory processes that lead to vasomotor symptoms. The fact that an increase in body temperature precedes most hot flushes is well known. This trigger initiates a series of heat-loss mechanisms, including cutaneous vasodilatation and subsequent flushing and sweating, which cause a slight drop in core body temperature and symptom relief. What induces a change in the thermoregulation set-point activity during the menopause is not known, but it may be mediated by a change in hormone concentrations that then affect brain neurotransmitters.

Hot flushes are associated with several biochemical changes, such as altered circulating concentrations of gonadal hormones, gonadotrophins and neurotransmitters. For example, circulating concentrations of luteinizing hormone, adrenocorticotrophic hormone and growth hormone increase before the hot flush and cortisone concentrations rise afterwards. Other associated hormone changes include a drop in mean concentrations of serum sex hormone binding globulin, an increase in the free androgen index and an increase in concentrations of calcitonin gene related peptide and neuropeptide Y. None, however, have ever been shown to initiate hot flushes.

What pathways are involved?

The direction of the thermoregulatory response could depend on direct or indirect stimulation of specific serotonin (5-HT) receptors in the brain. This could occur via modification of oestrogen levels.

Although several serotonin receptor families exist, the two 5-HT receptor subtypes believed to be most closely associated with temperature control are the serotonin 1a receptor ($5-HT1_A$) and the serotonin 2_A receptor ($5-HT2_A$, formerly known as 5-HT2). Administration of $5-HT2_A$ antagonists prevents hyperthermia in animal models of the serotonin syndrome, and direct stimulation of $5-HT2_A$ receptor induces hyperthermia in rodents. In contrast, peripheral administration of $5-HT1_A$ agonists to rodents and humans results in reductions in core body temperatures within

minutes. These data suggest that a balance between the $5-HT1_A$ and $5-HT2_A$ receptors might be important for optimum thermoregulation in mammals. The expression and activity of 5-HT receptors can be modulated by gonadal hormones and by adrenal corticosteroids, providing a functional link between serotonin and some of the hormonal systems linked to hot flushes. A recent hypothesis was that oestrogen withdrawal could be associated with a decline in circulating serotonin, thus increasing sensitivity of the hypothalamic $5HT2_A$ receptor. After an internal or an external stimulus, serotonin concentrations rise and the $5HT2_A$ receptor is stimulated (Figure 1). Consequently, a change in the thermoregulatory set-point occurs and a hot flush ensues.

Preclinical and clinical observations suggest cross-talk between gonadal hormones, especially oestrogen, and the thermoregulatory set-point. The set-point might be dependent on a balance of at least two serotonin receptors, and a change could induce vasomotor physiological responses to hot or cold stimuli to dissipate or preserve heat. How oestrogen affects this balance, and whether it acts directly or indirectly, is unknown.

Neurotransmitter modulators to treat hot flushes

Several agents have been used to treat hot flushes with various degrees of efficacy that, so

Table 1	
Role of different 5-HT receptors on temperature control. Adapted from Salmi and Ahlenius (1998).	
Receptor	**Role in temperature control**
$5-HT1_A$	• Agonists reduce body temperature and treat malignant hyperthermia
$5-HT2_A$	• Agonists reduce body temperature and treat malignant hyperthermia • Antagonists increase body temperature
$5-HT2_B$	• May have a role in temperature control but effect largely unknown

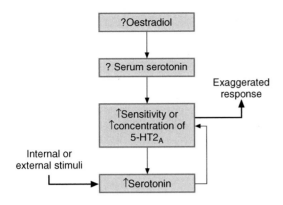

Figure 1
Hypothesis in genesis of hot flushes. Postmenopausal decrease in serum oestradiol decreases serum serotonin. This in turn increases the sensitivity of the 5-HT2$_A$ receptors. If a trigger stimuli occurs, such as an increase in external temperature, this will increase serotonin production that in turn will determine an exaggerated response because of upregulation of the receptor. Adapted from Berendsen (2000).

far, always have been inferior to the efficacy of oestrogen.

Clonidine

Clonidine, a centrally acting α-adrenoceptor agonist, originally was developed for the treatment of hypertension; it currently is used to treat hot flushes in women in whom HRT is contraindicated. Success is variable. Some authors have shown that clonidine reduces the number and intensity of hot flushes, whereas others failed to show a clear effect. One recent large placebo-controlled trial involving 194 postmenopausal women with breast cancer who were receiving adjuvant tamoxifen therapy showed that 0.1 mg/day clonidine was marginally superior to placebo in decreasing in hot flushes (38% versus 24%). The drug was generally well tolerated, and difficulty in sleeping was the most common side-effect.

Veralipride

Veralipride is a dopamine antagonist compound originally developed as a neuroleptic drug and then used for the relief of hot flushes in several countries. It is not available in the UK. Veralipride has been shown to be effective in reducing hot flushes, and in some studies effectiveness has paralleled that of oestrogen. However, several adverse effects, such as raised prolactin levels, rebound depression, and extrapyramidal side-effects, have been described with its use.

Selective serotonin reuptake inhibitors (SSRIs)

Given the possible role of serotonin in the pathogenesis of hot flushes, selective serotonin reuptake inhibitors (SSRIs) have been used to treat this symptom.

Venlafaxine

Venlafaxine is an antidepressant that inhibits the reuptake of both serotonin and noradrenaline. It reduces hot flushes in a dose-dependent manner: 37% with 37.5 mg/day venlafaxine and 61% with 75 mg/day and 150 mg/day. Dry mouth, decreased appetite, nausea and constipation were the reported side-effects. Venlafaxine also improved libido and mood. A similar effect on hot flushes was also found with other SSRIs: fluoxetine (20 mg/day), paroxetine (20 mg/day or 12.5 mg/day of the slow release formulation), trazodone (75 mg/day) and mirtazapine (30 mg/day).

Gabapentin

Gabapentin is a γ-aminobutyric acid analogue used to treat epilepsy, neurogenic pain and migraine. Case studies and a randomized, placebo–controlled study showed a 45% reduction in hot flushes in doses ranging from 300 mg/day to 1600 mg/day. Gabapentin also seems to be beneficial for women in whom aches, pains and paraesthesia are a significant feature of the climacteric syndrome. Tiredness seems to be the most common side-effect, particularly in the initial days of use. This may be avoided by gradually increasing the dose.

Conclusion

Drawbacks associated with hormonal treatments and the recognition of a neuroendocrinological cause for hot flushes has generated strategies that target adrenergic and neurosynaptic pathways. These agents at their best reduce hot flushes by 45–65%, which is far less that the 70–80% reduction achieved with oestrogen. They may be useful, however, in women who do not wish to or cannot take HRT. Further research on neurotransmitters will help to develop more appropriately targeted treatment strategies.

Further reading

Berendsen HHG. Hot flushes and serotonin. *J Br Menopause Soc* 2002; **8**; 30–4.

Berendsen HH, Weekers AH, Kloosterboer HJ. Effect of tibolone and raloxifene on the tail temperature of oestrogen-deficient rats. *Eur J Pharmacol* 2001; **419**: 47–54.

Casper RF, Graves GR, Reid RL. Objective measurement of hot flushes associated with the premenstrual syndrome. *Fertil Steril* 1987; **2**: 341–4.

Cryan JF, Kelliher P, Kelly JP, Leonard BE. Comparative effects of serotonergic agonists with varying efficacy at the 5-HT(1A) receptor on core body temperature: modification by the selective 5-HT(1A) receptor antagonist WAY 100635. *J Psychopharmacol* 1999; **13**: 278–3.

David A, Don R, Tajchner G, Weissglas L. Veralipride: alternative antidopaminergic treatment for menopausal symptoms. *Am J Obstet Gynecol* 1988; **158**: 1107–1.

Freedman RR. Biochemical, metabolic, and vascular mechanisms in menopausal hot flashes. *Fertil Steril* 1998; **70**: 332–7.

Freedman RR, Krell W. Reduced thermoregulatory null zone in postmenopausal women with hot flashes. *Am J Obstet Gynecol* 999; **181**: 66–70.

Guttuso T Jr, Kurlan R, McDermott MP, Kieburtz K. Gabapentin's effects on hot flashes in postmenopausal women: a randomized controlled trial. *Obstet Gynecol* 2003; **101**: 337–45.

Kronenberg F. Hot flashes: phenomenology, quality of life, and search for treatment options. *Exp Gerontol* 1994; **29**: 319–36

Loprinzi CL, Kugler JW, Sloan JA, et al. Venlafaxine in management of hot flashes in survivors of breast cancer: a randomised controlled trial. *Lancet* 2000; **356**: 2059–63

Pandya KJ, Raubertas RF, Flynn PJ, et al. Oral clonidine in postmenopausal patients with breast cancer experiencing tamoxifen-induced hot flashes: a University of Rochester Cancer Center Community Clinical Oncology Program study. *Ann Intern Med* 2000; **132**: 788–93.

Salmi P, Ahlenius S. Evidence for functional interactions between 5-HT1A and 5-HT2A receptors in rat thermoregulatory mechanisms. *Pharmacol Toxicol* 1998; **82**: 122–7.

Stearns V, Ullmer L, Lopez JF, et al. Hot flushes. *Lancet* 2002; **360**: 1851–61.

Verbeke K, Dhont M, Vandekerckhove D. Clinical and hormonal effects of long-term veralipride treatment in post-menopausal women. *Maturitas* 1988; **10**: 225–30.

5 Testosterone

Susan R Davis

Introduction

Many women complain of pervasive fatigue and loss of libido and sexual receptivity in the years approaching the menopause, during the transition and in the postmenopausal years. Clearly, multiple factors contribute to these symptoms, but a body of evidence suggests in some women they may in part be because of testosterone insufficiency. Testosterone therapy is used to varying degrees in different countries, and randomized controlled trials have now shown benefits for improved wellbeing and sexual satisfaction in women who are treated concurrently with testosterone and oestrogen therapy. The addition of testosterone also seems to improve bone density to a greater extent than oestrogen alone. At present, however, no data with respect to either safety or efficacy support the use of testosterone as a postmenopausal therapy alone.

Indications for the use of testosterone

Causes of low testosterone

No accepted definition of testosterone deficiency in women exists. Although the symptoms believed to characterize androgen insufficiency include low libido, dysphoric mood and persistent fatigue in women with adequate oestrogen, epidemiological data to support that these symptoms are related to low testosterone levels are lacking. Nor is there a clear cut parameter, such as a free testosterone level, with an accepted limit below which biochemical testosterone deficiency can be diagnosed. Other proposed features of testosterone insufficiency include vasomotor instability, vaginal dryness, decreased muscle strength and poor memory or cognitive function. Bone loss is also included as a potential part of the syndrome.

The adrenal glands produce the preandrogens androstenedione, dehydroepiandrosterone (DHEA) and DHEA sulphate, whereas the ovaries make androstenedione, DHEA and testosterone. About half of the circulating testosterone is produced by conversion of the preandrogens to testosterone, with androstenedione being the main precursor. Testosterone is metabolized in target organs and peripheral tissues to dihydrotestosterone (DHT) or is aromatized at these sites to oestradiol. Plasma levels of testosterone vary during the menstrual cycle, with the lowest levels during menstruation, and, as a result of production in the ovaries, they increase in the middle third of the menstrual cycle. This is followed by a second rise in production of androstenedione alone by the corpus luteum during the late luteal phase. Testosterone also exhibits a diurnal variation, with higher levels in the morning.

Under normal physiological conditions, only 1–2% of testosterone circulates unbound to plasma proteins. The rest is bound by sex hormone binding globulin (SHBG), which binds 66%, and albumin, which binds about 33%. Oestrogen and thyroxine increase concentrations of SHBG, which results in reduced levels of free testosterone; whereas elevated levels of testosterone, growth hormone and insulin reduce concentrations of SHBG, which results in increased absolute amounts of free testosterone. Total and free testosterone levels decline with age in premenopausal women from the early to mid reproductive years, remain stable across the menopausal transition and then remain stable or continue to decline with the gradual decline in adrenal function with increasing age. A recent clinical study has indicated that the postmenopausal ovary is not a significant source of androgens. This study, however, was conducted in women with adrenal insufficiency, so it may well be that lack of production of adrenal DHEAS, which

is an important precursor for ovarian androgen and oestrogen production, resulted in secondary low ovarian testosterone production.

Causes of androgen insufficiency

The proposed symptoms of androgen insufficiency are non-specific and may be caused by other conditions such as thyroid disease, anaemia and chronic fatigue. Depression and social and relationship problems may also present in a similar fashion. Conversely, these conditions may coexist with androgen insufficiency. Not uncommonly, women with low libido are depressed, and it may be difficult to determine whether depression causes low libido or vice versa.

Loss of ovarian function is the most clear-cut cause of diminished testosterone concentrations. After bilateral oophorectomy, an approximate 50% reduction in circulating testosterone levels occurs in premenopusal

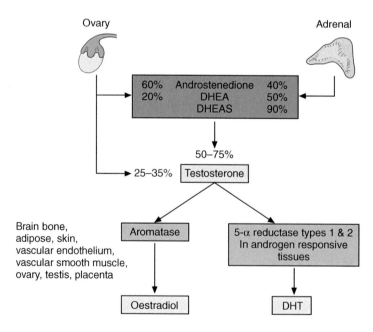

Figure 1
Testosterone production and metabolism.

women. Oophorectomized women more frequently report a worsening of their sexual life postoperatively than those who have undergone a hysterectomy alone or a natural spontaneous menopause. Some women after hysterectomy, with or without oophorectomy for benign disease, however, experience an improvement in sexual function – possibly because of a reduction in dyspareunia or menorrhagia. Conversely, some hysterectomized women undergo early ovarian failure, possibly because of disruption of ovarian blood flow at the time of hysterectomy, and subsequently experience a lowering of libido.

Other conditions that have been associated with low testosterone levels include adrenal failure, panhypopituitarism, premature menopause, human immunodeficiency virus wasting syndrome, systemic lupus erythematosus and rheumatoid arthritis.

Various drugs are associated with a decrease in circulating testosterone levels. These include exogenous oestrogens such as the oral contraceptive pill and oral postmenopausal hormone therapy. Exogenous oestrogens suppress pituitary luteinizing hormone production and thus reduce ovarian steroidogenesis. In addition, they increase concentrations of SHBG and consequently reduce the amount of free testosterone. Excessive thyroxine replacement can also potentially cause concentrations of SHBG to rise. Glucocorticoid therapy leads to suppression of adrenocorticotropic hormone and consequently to reduced adrenal production of androgens. Radiotherapy to the pelvis and chemotherapy may result in ovarian failure and hence lowered testosterone.

Measurement of testosterone

The diagnosis of testosterone insufficiency is one of exclusion and, when possible, demonstration of low free concentrations of testosterone. Total concentrations of testosterone, although the most common

measure for clinical studies, do not yield meaningful information about tissue exposure to androgens. Free testosterone is widely accepted as the strongest indicator of tissue exposure and variations in SHBG levels in women can have dramatic effects on free testosterone levels. No rapid, simple assay of total testosterone has been shown to produce reliable results in women with low to normal testosterone levels. The gold standard method for measurement of free testosterone is considered to be equilibrium dialysis. The Sodergard equation, however, can be used reliably to calculate free testosterone concentrations if concentrations of total testosterone, albumin and SHBG are known. Although this method needs reliable determination of total testosterone, this is more achievable in most laboratories than equilibrium dialysis.

Evidence of efficacy of testosterone therapy

Mood and sexuality

Several studies, including randomized controlled trials, have indicated a benefit of exogenous testosterone therapy in improving mood and well-being.

Clinical studies of supraphysiological testosterone therapy have shown improvements in sexual parameters in postmenopausal women. Less benefit has been seen with the addition of methyltestosterone, a non aromatizable androgen, to oestrogen therapy. The addition of testosterone undecanoate (40 mg/day), which raises testosterone levels into the supraphysiological range in a significant proportion of women, resulted in significant improvements. Frequency of satisfactory sexual activity, as well as increased sexual desire, has been shown in surgically menopausal women with a testosterone patch delivering 300 μg testosterone/day. With this dose, mean concentrations of free testosterone were close to the upper limit of the normal female range.

Bone

Osteoblasts possess androgen receptors, and androgens have been shown to directly stimulate bone cell proliferation and differentiation. Hyperandrogenic premenopausal women have higher bone mineral density (BMD), after correction for body mass index, than their normal female counterparts. Premenopausal women who experience bone loss confined to the hip have lower total and free testosterone concentrations (14% and 22% lower, respectively) than non-losers. Premenopausally, BMD also correlates strongly positively with body weight. Obesity suppresses SHBG with a resultant increase in free testosterone. This may partially explain the relation between obesity, free testosterone and increased BMD, with greater endogenous levels of biologically active free testosterone directly enhancing bone mass.

Studies of oral and parenteral oestrogen and oestrogen plus testosterone therapy in postmenopausal women have shown beneficial effects of testosterone on BMD and bone markers. Combined oestradiol and testosterone replacement with subcutaneous implant pellets increases hip and vertebral BMD in postmenopausal women, with the effects being greater than with oestradiol implants alone. No studies, however, have examined the effects on fracture. The latter is required before testosterone can be considered a valid treatment for osteoporosis.

Safety and side-effects

Excessive testosterone use will cause masculinization. Hirsutism, acne, temporal balding, voice deepening and clitoromegaly have not been increased significantly in recent studies of more physiological doses of parenteral testosterone therapy in women. Acne, however, has been reported with the use of combined esterified oestrogen and methyltestosterone. A modest increase in lean body mass, reduction in total body fat and no change in body mass index has been reported

with parenteral testosterone therapy. Oral methyltestosterone may decrease concentrations of triglycerides, HDL cholesterol and apolipoprotein A-1. Parenteral therapy, however, does not seem to have adverse lipid effects. Hepatocellular damage has been associated with high dose oral 17-α-alkylandrogens but not with standard female doses. Some studies imply an association with endogenous androgens and risk of breast cancer, but exogenous testosterone is associated with inhibition of oestrogen-induced mammary epithelial proliferation and suppression of oestrogen receptor expression.

Testosterone preparations

Oral

Testosterone is not readily bioavailable when administered orally, but it can be administered as methyltestosterone or testosterone undecanoate and results in a different metabolic profile, as described above. Methyltestosterone is believed not to be aromatized, thus its primary action is androgenic. Any potential beneficial effects of testosterone being aromatized to oestrogen peripherally thus are not apparent. Testosterone undecanoate is an oral formulation that is absorbed via the intestinal lymphatics and thus avoids the first pass effect in the liver. It has been approved for use in hypogonadal men, but there are neither efficacy nor safety data for women. The only available data in women indicate very variable serum concentrations.

Intramuscular

Intramuscular injections of 50–100 mg testosterone esters, each given 4–6 weeks apart, are used by some doctors. This may or may not result in a clinical response over 1–2 weeks or more. No pharmacokinetic or safety data are available for women. As peak levels are very superphysiological, this therapy should not be considered as a long-term treatment option.

Implants

In the UK, testosterone pellets have been approved for female use. These are implanted subcutaneously under local anaesthetic. A dose of 50 mg, obtained by cutting a 100 mg implant into half under sterile conditions, has been shown to be effective with a good safety profile. These implants remain effective for periods of 4–6 months. Repeat implantation should not be undertaken without confirming that total concentrations of testosterone corrected for SHBG or concentrations of free testosterone have declined into the lower quartile of the normal female range. The use of testosterone implants greater than 100 mg prudently would be avoided.

Future developments

The recent development of a transdermal testosterone matrix patch will provide yet another therapeutic option. The patch, which is now being investigated in clinical trials, delivers 300 µg/day. A transdermal patch will have some obvious advantages over oral and implant therapies. Women, however, may prefer to use a less apparent mode of replacement or may have difficulties with skin irritation or adhesion.

Other transdermal delivery systems for testosterone include a gel, a cream and a topical spray. Some pharmacists are also making available compounded creams and buccal lozenges. Pharmacokinetic data for these individualized preparations are lacking, however, and clinical trials of their use have not been published.

Contraindications to testosterone

Testosterone is contraindicated for women who are pregnant, lactating, have the potential of conceiving or have a known or suspected androgen-dependent neoplasm. A current or past history of acne, hirsutism or androgenic alopecia also are strong contraindications. It is

the author's experience that caution also should be exercised for women who have central obesity and low concentrations of SHBG and/or insulin resistance with low concentrations of SHBG, as standard testosterone therapy is likely to result in very high concentrations of free testosterone and thus carry a greater risk of side-effects. All postmenopausal women given testosterone therapy should be using concurrent oestrogen therapy. No clinical data are available about the use of testosterone in postmenopausal women who are not taking oestrogen; however, such use may well result in adverse metabolic and cosmetic side-effects.

Conclusion

Substantial evidence from randomized controlled trials now shows that testosterone therapy will improve sexual satisfaction and mood in surgically menopausal women treated with concurrent oestrogen, with less data in naturally menopausal women and premenopausal women. Long-term safety data for combined oestrogen–testosterone therapy are lacking, however, and the effects of testosterone-only therapy in postmenopausal women are unknown. Although there seems to be considerable potential for testosterone to improve the quality of life for selected women, inappropriate and/or excessive use of testosterone carries the risk of masculinization and possibly more serious side-effects. All women treated with testosterone need to be carefully monitored both biochemically and clinically, and they should have long-term follow-up for adverse sequelae.

Further reading

Bachmann GA, Bancroft J, Braunstein G, et al. Female androgen insufficiency: the Princeton Consensus Statement on definition, classification and assessment. Fertil Steril 2002; 77: 665.

Buckler HM, McElhone K, Durrington PN, et al. The effects of low-dose testosterone treatment on lipid metabolism, clotting factors and ultrasonographic ovarian morphology in women. Clin Endocrinol (Oxf) 1998; 49: 173–8.

Couzinet B, Meduri G, Lecce M, et al. The post menopausal ovary is not a major androgen producing gland. *J Clin Endocrinol Metab* 2001; **86**: 5060–5.

Davis SR. Androgen replacement in women: a commentary. *J Clin Endocrinol Metab* 1999; **84**: 1886–91.

Davis SR. The use of testosterone after menopause. *J Br Menopause Soc* 2004 (in press).

Davis S, Rees M, Ribot J, et al. Efficacy and safety of testosterone patches for the treatment of low sexual desire in surgically menopausal women. Abstract presented at the *59th Annual Meeting of the American Society for Reproductive Medicine, San Antonio, Texas, 11–15 October 2003*.

Davis SR, Walker KZ, Strauss BJ. Effects of estradiol with and without testosterone on body composition and relationships with lipids in post-menopausal women. *Menopause* 2000; **7**: 395–401.

Floter A, Nathorst-Boos J, Carlstrom K, von Schoultz B. Addition of testosterone to estrogen replacement therapy in oophorectomized women: effects on sexuality and well-being. *Climacteric* 2002; **5**: 357–65.

Goldstat R, Briganti E, Tran J, et al. Transdermal testosterone improves mood, well being and sexual function in premenopausal women. *Menopause* 2003; **10**: 390–8.

Klee GG, Heser D. Techniques to measure testosterone in the elderly. *Mayo Clinic Proceedings* 2000; **75**: S19–25.

Laughlin G.A, Barrett-Connor E, Kritz-Silverstein D, Von Muhlen D. Hysterectomy, oophorectomy, and endogenous sex hormone levels in older women: the Rancho Bernardo Study. *J Clin Endocrinol Metab* 2000; **85**: 645–51.

Lobo R, Rosen RC, Yang H-M, et al. Comparative effects of oral esterified estrogens with and without methyl testosterone on endocrine profiles and dimensions of sexual function in postmenopausal women with hypoactive sexual desire. *Fertil Steril* 2003; **79**: 1341–52.

Miller K, Sesmilo G, Schiller A, et al. Androgen deficiency in women with hypopituitarism. *J Clin Endocrinol Metab* 2001; **86**: 561–7.

Savvas M, Studd JWW, Norman S, et al. Increase in bone mass after one year of percutaneous oestradiol and testosterone implants in post menopausal women who have previously received long-term oral oestrogens. *Br J Obstet Gynaecol* 1992; **99**: 757–60.

Shifren JL, Braunstein G, Simon J, et al. Transdermal testosterone treatment in women with impaired sexual function after oophorectomy. *N Engl J Med* 2000; **343**: 682–8.

Zhou J, Ng S, Adesanya-Famuiya O, et al. Testosterone inhibits estrogen-induced mammary epithelial proliferation and suppresses estrogen receptor expression. *FASEB J* 2000; **14**: 1725–30.

6 Urinary incontinence

Andrew Sinclair and Andrew Hextall

Introduction

Urinary incontinence is a common problem, which although not life threatening, may have an adverse effect on the quality of life of adult women of all ages. Epidemiological studies have shown that 70% of postmenopausal women with incontinence relate the onset of their urinary symptoms to their final menstrual period, with 20% of women attending a menopause clinic complaining of urgency and 50% suffering from stress incontinence. The use of oestrogen replacement therapy to treat bladder symptoms has been controversial for many years and was assessed recently in a Cochrane review. For many women, alternative therapies will be more effective and acceptable.

Simple assessment

Most patients with incontinence will have a number of different urinary symptoms, but the most common problems are stress and/or urge incontinence. Considerable overlap exists between the two conditions: some women with stress incontinence complain of frequency and urgency, while often women with urgency will also leak when coughing or during exercise. The patient's most bothersome symptoms usually can be determined very quickly. Urinary tract infection also is a common complaint in postmenopausal women – mainly because of an increase in uropathogens in the vaginal flora associated with oestrogen deficiency.

After a simple history is taken and an examination is performed, urinalysis is useful to exclude blood or glucose in the urine and may give an indication that infection may be found on culture of a midstream specimen. A postmicturition residual estimation with ultrasound will exclude significant voiding difficulties. Bladder diaries are an excellent tool for obtaining an objective estimation of fluid intake and voiding patterns. Many women will be found to be not drinking enough or consuming an excessive amount: often of tea or fizzy drinks that may irritate the bladder. Most patients with urinary symptoms should be advised to drink about 1500–2000 ml per 24 hours, although those with recurrent infections may need larger volumes.

Conservative treatments can be initiated on the basis of the patient's symptoms, but the current consensus is for urodynamic studies always to be performed whenever surgery is contemplated, so that a definitive diagnosis can be made; although this approach has not been tested in robust randomized studies. Urodynamics are also useful when the underlying problem is unclear from the patient's history or when first line treatment has not been successful. Videourodynamics provides additional information, but it is not necessary in every case. Magnetic resonance imaging and ultrasound scanning have given insights into the pathophysiology of incontinence, but they have yet to be used widely outside of a research setting.

Stress incontinence

Stress urinary incontinence is the complaint of involuntary leakage on effort or exertion or on sneezing or coughing. The aetiology is multifactorial and includes pregnancy and childbirth, pelvic surgery, ageing and disorders of collagen structure and metabolism. The peak prevalence occurs around the age of the menopause (Figure 1), and so oestrogen deficiency has been implicated as a risk factor for some women.

Conservative treatment

Physiotherapy is the first line treatment for urinary stress incontinence and includes a package of care, the main component being pelvic floor exercises, which were first proposed by Kegel in 1948. Many women with stress incontinence will improve quickly as they regain 'the knack' of contracting their pelvic floor, while others will take longer to develop the bulk and tone of their musculature. Pelvic floor exercises provide symptomatic improvement in up to 70% of women as long as they perform them properly and for a prolonged period of time. The highest success rates are often seen in well motivated patients who are instructed by a specialist physiotherapist and are prepared to continue with exercises in the long term. Adjuvant therapies such as electrical stimulation or vaginal cones may also be useful, but they have been shown to be less effective than pelvic floor exercises.

Medical management

Oral α-adrenergic agonists, such as phenylpropanolamine, increase the maximum urethral closure pressure and therefore have been used, sometimes in combination with oestrogen, to treat urinary stress incontinence. Unfortunately, low cure rates and significant side-effect profiles make these drugs less than ideal agents, and they no longer should be used for this indication.

More recently, the serotonin/noradrenaline reuptake inhibitor duloxetine hydrochloride has been used in a phase 3 trial of women with stress incontinence. The study showed a 50% reduction in incontinence episodes with duloxetine compared with 27% with placebo.

Surgical management

At least 100 operations are described for urinary stress incontinence, but unfortunately

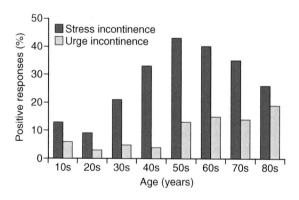

Figure 1
Changes in prevalence of stress and urge incontinence with increasing age among 1100 women. Adapted from Kondo *et al* (1990).

none have a 100% success rate without complications. In general, surgery is reserved for women who have failed to respond adequately to conservative measures and in whom urodynamic studies show a stable bladder. It is important to choose the correct procedure for each patient at the outset, as the first operation performed usually has the best chance of success. Many techniques can be performed under local or regional anaesthetic, resulting in a reduced hospital stay and a quicker return to normal activities.

Burch colposuspension
Burch colposuspension remains the 'gold standard' against which all others are compared. The procedure normally is carried out under general anaesthesia and has an accepted cure rate of >90% at one year and 69% at 10 years for women who have not had previous surgery. The recovery period is long, however, and complications include the development of voiding difficulties (10–20%) and detrusor overactivity (15%), as well as the long-term risk of prolapse.

Tension free vaginal tape
The tension free vaginal tape (TVT) procedure was first introduced in Scandinavia during 1994–1995, and it can be carried out under local or regional anaesthesia with a short hospital stay (often as day case surgery). With the patient in the lithotomy position, a small longitudinal incision is made in the vagina at the level of the midurethra, with two further 1 cm incisions in the skin over the pubic bone. Specially designed needles are used to pass a polypropylene tape through the vagina and behind the pubic bone on either side of the urethra, so that the tape lies loosely under the midportion of the urethra to form a sling (Figure 2). Bladder perforation occurs in about 4% of cases, but as a cystoscopy is performed during the procedure, this should be recognized immediately and rectified by passage of the needles more laterally, without further consequence. A recently reported randomized study showed that TVT had similar short-term

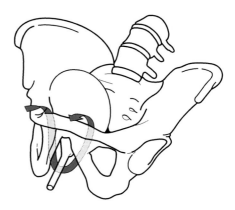

Figure 2
Tension free vaginal tape (TVT) procedure used to treat urinary stress incontinence. The tape is seen to be placed under the mid-urethra. The procedure has an 85–90% cure rate.

success rates to colposuspension but with a much quicker recovery period. In addition, the National Institute for Clinical Excellence (NICE) in the UK found the procedure to be more cost effective. However, the lack of long-term data and concerns about rejection of the tape material remain.

Urethral bulking agents
Urethral bulking agents are useful in elderly patients, particularly if the vagina is shortened or scarred by previous surgery, which makes more major procedures difficult. A number of different substances have been used, including paraffin, cartilage and autologous fat, but in the UK, the most popular bulking agents currently in use are glutaraldehyde cross-linked (GAX) collagen and macroplastique, which consists of vulcanized silicone rubber particles suspended in a non-silicone carrier gel. Short-term subjective cure rates of 50% are typical, with the objective results usually lower, but after five years, as few as 20% of women will still be continent. Several injections may be necessary, but most injections can be

performed under local anaesthetic with a quick recovery and a low risk of complications. Although overall treatment costs are lower than for most major procedures, injectable agents are very expensive, which limits their use.

Urge urinary incontinence

Urge urinary incontinence is the complaint of involuntary leakage accompanied by or immediately preceded by urgency. The most common cause of urge incontinence is detrusor overactivity; however, a postmenopausal woman may develop urinary urgency for a number of other reasons (Box 1). Investigation often is needed to make an accurate diagnosis. Urodynamic studies are also helpful and may show the presence of involuntary bladder contractions during the filling phase, which may be phasic or provoked – perhaps by listening to running water or washing hands. Cystoscopy may be necessary if malignancy is suspected or if the patient has recurrent infections.

Box 1
Common causes of postmenopausal urgency.
- Detrusor overactivity
- Impaired emptying
- Prolapse
- Atrophic vaginitis
- Chronic cystitis or recurrent infections
- Excessive fluid intake
- Medical conditions: for example, diabetes
- Drug therapy: for example, diuretics

Conservative treatment

Several behavioural modifications can help with urge incontinence. Changes in fluid intake are often necessary, and bladder diaries sometimes are useful to illustrate this. For those who go to the toilet infrequently, timed voiding (perhaps every two hours) may be necessary to help prevent the bladder becoming excessively full. However, most women will go to the toilet

frequently and bladder retraining – gradually increasing the time between voids – may lead to short-term subjective and objective improvements. Further benefit may be gained from pelvic floor physiotherapy and distraction techniques. Unfortunately, the relapse rate is disappointingly high, and for many women, detrusor overactivity may lead to long-term urinary symptoms despite the use of behavioural and other therapies.

Medical management

Most people who seek medical advice for urge incontinence will at some point try anticholinergic therapy. A recent meta-analysis suggested that the benefit of this type of treatment over placebo may be small and of questionable significance. Despite this finding, many women in clinical practice do seem to have a reduction in the frequency and severity of urge incontinence episodes at least in the short term. However, side-effects, such as dry mouth, bloating and constipation significantly affect compliance with treatment. A number of preparations are available; the most commonly prescribed are tolterodine, oxybutynin and trospium chloride.

Tolterodine

Tolterodine is a competitive muscarinic receptor antagonist with selectivity for M_3 receptors in the bladder. In a recent study, 1529 patients (80% women) with urinary frequency and urgency were randomized to once daily tolterodine extended release (ER), twice daily tolterodine immediate release (IR) or placebo for 12 weeks. The median reduction in urge incontinence episodes was 71% for tolterodine ER, 60% for tolterodine IR and 33% for placebo. In addition to improved efficacy, tolterodine ER also had a lower incidence of dry mouth (23% overall but considered severe in only 1.8% of patients).

Oxybutynin

Oxybutynin is a tertiary amine with high affinity for muscarinic receptors in both the bladder and salivary glands. Although as efficacious as tolterodine, oxybutynin produces significant problems with mouth dryness and other side-effects, such that less than 20% of women continued with the immediate-release formulation for more than six months. A controlled-release formulation that may prove more acceptable in the long term has been produced. In a randomized study, significant reductions in urinary urge incontinence episodes were seen in women who took controlled release oxybutynin (mean decrease 83%) and immediate-release oxybutynin (mean decrease 76%). The incidence of dry mouth was dose-dependent in both groups, but significantly fewer women who took the controlled-release oxybutynin considered the symptom of dry mouth to be moderate or severe.

Trospium chloride

Trospium chloride is a quaternary ammonium compound that non-selectively blocks muscarinic receptors. Drug interactions are minimal, so this preparation may be useful for women already taking other medications. In addition, very little trospium crosses the blood–brain barrier, so problems with headache are rare. Overall efficacy is similar to that with tolterodine and oxybutynin, but trospium currently is available only in a twice-daily formulation.

Unfortunately, despite trying a number of different preparations, for many women the symptoms resulting from detrusor overactivity may lead to significant morbidity over many years.

Surgical management

Continence surgery rarely is indicated for the treatment of urge incontinence secondary to detrusor overactivity. It usually is reserved for those patients with severe problems who have failed to respond to all conservative and medical treatments. Sacral nerve stimulation and neuromodulation is a useful alternative to

surgery in selected patients, but the treatment is expensive and at present is available only in a small number of centres.

Women with mixed incontinence (involuntary leakage associated with urgency and also with exertion, effort, sneezing or coughing) may benefit from surgery but usually only when detrusor overactivity has been treated effectively. Even in this situation, success rates are lower than for surgery for pure urodynamic stress incontinence, and a small number of women may be left with intractable urge leakage.

Conclusion

Urinary symptoms are common in postmenopausal women and can have a significant impact on quality of life. Many patients can be treated effectively after basic assessment with simple measures, such as fluid modification, bladder retraining and pelvic floor physiotherapy. For women with stress incontinence who do not improve sufficiently with pelvic floor exercises, a number of effective surgical options are available, with tension free vaginal tape (TVT) the most popular at present. Urinary urgency after the menopause has many causes, and investigation may be necessary to make an accurate diagnosis. Detrusor overactivity seems to improve in most women with anticholinergic drugs, but it may be necessary to try a number of different preparations, and the long-term benefits are unclear.

Further reading

Abrams P, Blaivas JG, Fowler CJ, et al. The role of neuromodulation in the management of urinary urge incontinence. BJU Int 2003; 91: 355–9.

Abrams P, Cardozo L, Fall M, et al. The standardization of terminology in lower urinary tract function: report from the standardization sub-committee of the International Continence Society. Urology 2003; 61: 37–49.

Abrams P, Freeman RN, Anderstrom C, Mattiasson A. Efficacy and tolerability of tolterodine compared to oxybutynin and placebo in patients with detrusor instability. J Urol 1997; 157: 103.

Alcalay M, Monga A, Stanton SL. Burch colposuspension: a 10–20 year follow up. *Br J Obstet Gynaecol* 1995; **102**: 740–5.

Anderson KE, Appell R, Cardozo LD, *et al.* The pharmacological treatment of urinary incontinence. *BJU Int* 1999; **84**: 923–47.

Blackwell AL, Moore KH. Does detrusor overactivity ever cease? Repeat urodynamic testing at 1 to 9 years. *Neurourol Urodyn* 2003; **22**: 462–3.

Bo K, Talseth T, Holme I. Single blind, randomized controlled trial of pelvic floor exercises, electrical stimulation, vaginal cones, and no treatment in management of genuine stress incontinence in women. *BMJ* 1999; **318**: 487–93.

Cardozo L, Chapple CR, Toozs-Hobson P, *et al.* Efficacy of trospium chloride in patients with detrusor instability: a placebo-controlled, randomised, double blind, multicentre clinical trial. *BJU Int* 2000; **85**: 659–64.

Cardozo L, Tapp A, Versi E. The lower urinary tract in peri and post-menopausal women. In Samsioe G, Bonne Erickson P, eds. *The urogenital oestrogen deficiency syndrome*. Bagsverd: Novo Industri AS, 1987: 10–17.

Fantl JA, Wyman JF, McClish DK, *et al.* Efficacy of bladder training in older women with urinary incontinence. *JAMA* 1991; **265**: 609–13.

National Institute of Clinical Excellence. *Guidance on the use of tension-free vaginal tape (Gynecare TVT) for stress incontinence. Technology appraisal 56.* London: NICE, 2003.

Herbison P, Hay-Smith J, Ellis G, Moore K. Effectiveness of anticholinergic drugs compared with placebo in the treatment of overactive bladder: systematic review. *BMJ* 2003; **326**: 841–4.

Herzog AR, Fultz NG, Brock BM, Brown MB. Urinary incontinence and psychological distress among older adults. *Psychol Aging* 1988; **3**: 115–21.

Hextall A, Cardozo L. Effects during the lifecycle (menopause). In: Cardozo L, Staskin D, eds. *Textbook of female urology and urogynaecology.* London: Isis Medical Media Limited, 2001: 994–1006.

Holmes DM, Stone AR, Bary PR, *et al.* Bladder retraining: 3 years on. *Br J Urol* 1983; **55**: 660–4.

Kegel AH. Progressive resistance exercise in the functional restoration of the perineal muscles. *Am J Obstet Gynecol* 1948; **56**: 238–49.

Kondo A, Kato K, Saito M, *et al.* Prevalence of hand washing incontinence in females in comparison with stress and urge incontinence. *Neurourol Urodyn* 1990; **9**: 330–1.

Minassian VA, Drutz HP, Al-Badr A. Urinary incontinence as a worldwide problem. *Int J Gynaecol Obstet* 2003; **82**: 327–38.

Moehrer B, Hextall A, Jackson S. Oestrogens for urinary incontinence in women (Cochrane review). In: *The Cochrane Library, Issue 1, 2004.* Chichester: John Wiley, 2004.

Van Kerrebroeck P, Kreder K, Jonas U, *et al.* Tolterodine once-daily: superior efficacy and tolerability in the treatment of overactive bladder. *Urology* 2001; **57**: 414–21.

Versi E, Appell R, Mobley D, *et al.* Dry mouth with conventional and controlled release oxybutynin in urinary incontinence. The Ditropan XL study group. *Obstet Gynecol* 2000; **95**: 718–21.

Ward K, Hilton P. Prospective multicentre randomized trail of tension-free vaginal tape and colposuspension as primary treatment for stress incontinence. *BMJ* 2002; **325**: 67–70.

Alternative and complementary therapies

Herbal medicine

Alyson Huntley and Joanna Thompson Coon

Introduction

The use of herbal remedies is prevalent among women seeking relief from menopausal symptoms (Figure 1). A survey conducted in the USA (397 women approaching or in menopause recruited from primary care centres) found that 25% had used one of four herbal preparations (phytoestrogens, *Hypericum perforatum*, *Ginkgo biloba* or *Panax ginseng*) in the previous six months, and 68% of them reported that the herbal product improved their symptoms. In the UK, 31% of the adult population reported ever having used over the counter herbal remedies, with 20% reporting use in the previous 12 months (1997–1998). Use of herbal remedies was significantly more popular with women than with men (33% *vs* 12%; *p* value <0.001).

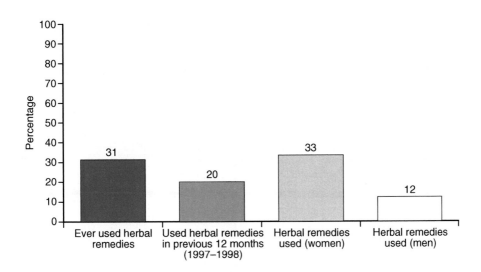

Figure 1
Use of herbal remedies in the UK.

Actaea racemosa (black cohosh)

Actaea racemosa (formerly known as Cimicifuga racemosa), a herbaceous perennial plant native to North America, is widely used to alleviate menopausal symptoms. Early animal studies suggest an 'oestrogen-like' activity; more recent work suggests the effects may be due to a central activity.

Five randomized clinical trials of A. racemosa are available in the literature. Two trials had poor methods, being of open design with no placebo group, and extrapolation of these results therefore is difficult. The results from two trials with better methods are promising. In a study of 80 postmenopausal women (at least three hot flushes per day with one other symptom, such as sweating or palpitations) who received treatment with A. racemosa (80 mg/day), conjugated equine oestrogen (0.625 mg/day) or identical placebo for 12 weeks, improvements were seen in the Kupperman index and Hamilton anxiety scale in all groups. The greatest improvement was seen in those who took A. racemosa, but differences between groups were not significant. Wuttke et al treated 62 postmenopausal women (at least three hot flushes per day, follicle stimulating hormone (FSH) ≥25mU/ml and amenorrhoea for >6 months) with an A. racemosa preparation (40 mg/day), conjugated equine oestrogens (0.625 mg/day) or matching placebo for 12 weeks. No significant differences were seen in

the reductions of menopause symptoms between groups, although trends for greater improvements were seen with A. racemosa and the conjugated oestrogen preparation compared with placebo (Figure 2).

A placebo controlled trial of 85 female survivors of breast cancer predominantly treated with concomitant tamoxifen found no significant difference in the reduction of hot flushes between those treated with A. racemosa (40mg/day) and those who took placebo.

A systematic review of the safety of A. racemosa preparations concluded that when taken for a limited period, a slight risk of mild, transient adverse events exists. More serious adverse events seem to be rare. The often limited data available means it is difficult to ascertain causality with the A. racemosa preparation. Several case reports have noted hepatitis associated with the ingestion of A. racemosa, but again a definitive assessment of causality is difficult to achieve. Little data are available about the long-term use of A. racemosa, particularly with respect to endometrial or breast tissue stimulation.

Piper methysticum (kava kava)

In the South Pacific, extracts from the rhizome P. methysticum have been used for recreational and medicinal purposes for thousands of years.

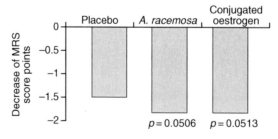

p values compared to placebo

Figure 2
The effect of A. racemosa on menopause symptoms. Adapted from Wuttke et al 2003.

A Cochrane review concluded that *P. methysticum* extract may be an effective symptomatic treatment option for anxiety. Concern about the number of possible cases of liver damage associated with the ingestion of *P. methysticum*, however, has lead regulatory authorities in the USA, Canada, Australia and UK to suspend or withdraw *P. methysticum* products from the market pending further evidence of their safety.

Four randomized clinical trials have investigated the role of *P. methysticum* in the management of menopausal symptoms. In two of the trials, although improvements in various endpoints were seen after treatment with *P. methysticum*, no comparisons were made with placebo. Interpretation of these results thus is difficult. In the two remaining trials, treatment with *P. methysticum* seemed to be promising. Warnecke randomized 40 menopausal women to receive either *P. methysticum* extract (300 mg/day) or placebo for eight weeks. Scores on the Kupperman index and Hamilton anxiety scale were significantly better with *P. methysticum* compared with placebo at weeks 1, 4 and 8. In an open study that investigated the effect of calcium and *P. methysticum* extract on mood, Cagnacci et al randomized 68 perimenopausal women (amenorrhoea for 6–24 months, at least

three hot flushes per day and follicle stimulating hormone >30 IU/l) to receive *P. methysticum* (100 or 200 mg/day) or no treatment for 12 weeks. All women also received calcium supplementation (1 g/day). Anxiety was evaluated with the state trait anxiety inventory, depression by the Zung scale and climacteric symptoms by the Greene scale. Improvements were seen in all three measures in both groups; however, only the decline in anxiety induced by *P. methysticum* was significantly greater than that spontaneously occurring in control women.

Oenothera biennis (evening primrose)

Oil derived from the seeds of *O. biennis* is a rich source of γ linolenic acid. In the only available randomized, placebo-controlled trial, 56 menopausal women (at least three hot flushes per day, raised concentrations of FSH and/or amenorrhoea for at least six months) were randomized to receive 'evening primrose oil' (4000 mg/day) or placebo (liquid paraffin) for 24 weeks. Unfortunately, only 35 women completed the trial (18 who took 'evening primrose oil' and 17 who took placebo); in all cases, the decision to withdraw was based on a perception of a poor clinical response to

Anxiety scores	0 month	1 month	3 months
Control group	48±1.6	48±1.0	47.8±1.8
Kava group combined 100 & 200 mg plus Ca	46.5±1.5	43.1±1.3*	41.9±1.4

* p<0.0001 compared to control

Depression scores	0 month	1 month	3 months
Control group	25±2.3	24.8±2.4	23.6±2.4
Kava group combined 100 & 200 mg plus Ca	27.5±1.6	24.63±1.8*	21.85±1.3

* p<0.0006 compared to control

Figure 3
Effect of calcium and *P. methysticum* extract on mood. Adapted from Cagnacci et al 2003.

treatment. No significant differences in the frequency of hot flushes between groups were observed, which indicates that 'evening primrose oil' offered no benefit over placebo.

The oil derived from *O. biennis* seeds seems to be safe, with adverse events limited to headache, nausea and diarrhoea.

Angelica sinensis (dong quai)

The root of *Angelica sinensis*, a fragrant perennial plant native to southwest China, is one of the oldest and most established agents used in traditional Chinese medicine. It is most commonly available commercially as a component of combination preparations. One randomized clinical trial of an extract of the crushed root of *A. sinensis* used alone is available. Hirata and colleagues randomized 71 postmenopausal women (amenorrhoea for >6 months, more than five troublesome night sweats or vasomotor flushes per week and follicle stimulating hormone <30 mIU/mL) to receive *A. sinensis* powder or placebo (maltodextrin) for 24 weeks. Although improvements on the Kupperman index and daily flush diary were seen in symptoms in both groups compared with baseline, no evidence suggested that *A. sinensis* was superior to placebo in relieving symptoms. In addition, no differences were seen in endometrial thickness or vaginal maturation between groups.

Case reports suggest that *A. sinensis* may cause bleeding when administered in conjunction with warfarin and it may be associated with photosensitization reactions.

Ginkgo biloba (ginkgo)

Systematic and Cochrane reviews suggest beneficial effects with *G. biloba* in cognitive impairment and dementia. One randomized clinical trial of the effects of treatment with *G. biloba* on cognition and mood in postmenopausal women is available. Hartley *et al* randomized 34 postmenopausal women

(53–65 years, amenorrhoea for >12 months) to seven days' treatment with *G. biloba* or placebo. A battery of cognitive tests, measurements of mood and the Greene climacteric scale were administered before and after treatment. *G. biloba* was associated with better performances in tests of non-verbal memory, frontal lobe function and sustained attention. No significant differences were seen between groups in immediate or delayed paragraph recall, delayed recall of pictures, menopausal symptoms, sleepiness, bodily symptoms or aggression.

G. biloba extracts seem to be relatively safe, with most reported adverse events being mild and benign. Several case reports have linked *G. biloba* extracts with bleeding episodes; however, given the widespread use of these products worldwide, this seems to be a relatively rare phenomenon.

Panax ginseng (ginseng)

Panax ginseng, a perennial herb native to Korea and China, has been used as an herbal remedy in eastern Asia for thousands of years. Modern therapeutic claims refer to vitality, immune function, cancer, cardiovascular disease and improvement of cognitive, physical and sexual function. Wiklund *et al* investigated the effects of a standardized *P. ginseng* extract on 384 postmenopausal women (at least six episodes of hot flushes during at least three of the past seven days and amenorrhoea for >6 months) in a randomized placebo-controlled 16-week study. The psychological general wellbeing score (PGWB) and the women's health questionnaire (WHQ) were used to assess the effects of *P. ginseng* on quality of life. Significant differences were seen for the depression, wellbeing and health subscales of the PGWB in favour of *P. ginseng*. No other significant differences between treatment groups were seen, although a considerable decrease in symptoms was seen in both groups. No changes in the levels of oestradiol and FSH, endometrial thickness, vaginal pH or vaginal cytology values were observed compared with baseline.

A systematic review of the safety of *P. ginseng* concluded that it is well tolerated by most users, with the most frequently observed adverse events being mild and reversible. Several case reports, however, link the ingestion of 'ginseng' with postmenopausal bleeding and mastalgia; herb–drug interactions have been observed with warfarin, phenelzine and alcohol.

Herbal combinations

Several randomized clinical trials have looked at herbal combinations for menopausal symptoms. Results of these are difficult to extrapolate, as they refer to single trials with defined herbal mixtures. Positive results were seen in a trial of the combination of *A. racemosa* and *Hypericum perforatum*, although the improvements were not considered to be clinically relevant. In placebo-controlled trials of herbal mixtures of *Arctium lappa, Glycyrrhiza glabra, Leonorus cardiaca, Angelica sinensis* and *Dioscorea barbasco, Rehmannia glutinosa, Cornus officinalis, Dioscorea opposita, Alisma orientalis, Paeonia suffruticosa, Poria cocos, Citrus reticulata, Lycium chinensis, Albizzia julibrissin, Zizphus jujba, Eclipta prostrata* and *Ligustrum lucidum*, and a cream containing *Dioscorea vilosa, Linum usitatissimum, Pelargonium graveolen* and *Salvia officinalis*, although improvements were seen in both groups (placebo and verum) no intergroup differences were found.

Further reading

Boblitz N, Schrader E, Henneicke-von Zepelin H-H, Wüstenberg P. Benefit of a fixed drug combination containing St John's Wort and Black Cohosh for climacteric patients – results of a randomised clinical trial. *Focus Altern Complement Ther* 1999; **5**: 85–6.

Boon H, Smith M. *The botanical pharmacy*. Ontario: Quarry Press Inc, 1999.

Borrelli F, Izzo AA, Ernst E. Pharmacological effects of *Cimicifuga racemosa*. *Life Sci* 2003; **73**: 1215–29.

Cagnacci A, Arangino S, Renzi A, *et al.* Kava-Kava administration reduces anxiety in perimenopausal women. *Maturitas* 2003; **44**: 103–9.

Dailey RK, Neale AV, Northrup J, *et al.* Herbal product use and menopause symptom relief in primary care patients: a MetroNet study. *J Women's Health* 2003; **12**: 633–41.

Davis SR, Briganti EM, Chen RQ, *et al.* The effects of Chinese medicinal herbs on postvasomotor symptoms of Australian women. *Med J Aust* 2001; **174**: 68–71.

Hartley DE, Heinze L, Elsabagh S, File SE. Effects on cognition and mood in postmenopausal women of 1-week treatment with *Ginkgo biloba*. *Pharmacol Biochem Behaviour* 2003; **75**: 711–20.

Hirata JD, Small R, Swiersz LM, *et al.* Does Dong Quai have estrogenic effects in postmenopausal women? A double-blind, placebo controlled trial. *Fertil Steril* 1997; **68**: 981–7.

Hudson TS, Standish L, Breed C, *et al.* Clinical and endocrinological effects of a menopausal botanical formula. *J Naturopath Med* 1999; **7**: 73–7.

Huntley A, Ernst E. A systematic review of the safety of black cohosh. *Menopause* 2003; **10**: 58–64.

Komesaroff PA, Black CVS, Cable V, Sudhir K. Effects of wild yam extract on menopausal symptoms, lipids and sex hormones in healthy menopausal women. *Climacteric* 2001; **4**: 144–50.

Laino C. Black cohosh linked to autoimmune hepatitis. New York: Medscape, 2003 (http://www medscape com/viewarticle/463059).

Pittler MH, Ernst E. Kava extract for treating anxiety (Cochrane Review). In: *The Cochrane Library, Issue 4, 2003*. Chichester: John Wiley: CD003383.

Stoll W. Phytotherapeutikum beeinflußt atrophisches Vaginalepithel. Doppelblindversuch Cimicifuga vs Östrogenpräparat. (Phytotherapeutic effect on vaginal epithelium atrophy: a double blind study of Cimifuga vs. oestrogens.) *Therapeutikon* 1987; **1**: 23–31 (in German).

Thomas KJ, Nicholl JP, Coleman P. Use and expenditure on complementary medicine in England: a population based survey. *Complement Ther Med* 2001; **9**: 2–11.

Thompson Coon J, Ernst E. Panax ginseng: a systematic review of adverse effects and drug interactions. *Drug Safety* 2002; **25**: 323–44.

Warnecke G. Psychosomatische Dysfunktionen im weiblichen Klimakterium. Klinische Wirksamkeit und Verträglichkeit von Kava-Extrakt WS 1490. (Neurovegetative dystonia in the female climacteric. Studies on the clinical efficacy and tolerance of kava extract WS1490.) *Fortschritte Medizin* 1991; **4**: 3–7 (in German).

Whiting PW, Clouston A, Kerlin P. Black cohosh and other herbal remedies associated with acute hepatitis. *Med J Aust* 2002; **177**: 432–5.

Wiklund IK, Mattsson L-A, Lindgren R, Limoni C, for the Swedish Alternative Medicine Group. Effects of a standardised ginseng extract on quality life and physiological parameters in symptomatic postmenopausal women: a double blind, placebo controlled trial. *Int J Clin Pharm Res* 1999; **XIX**: 89–99.

Wuttke W, Seidlova-Wuttke D, Gorkow C. The *Cimicifuga* preparation BNO 1055 vs. conjugated estrogens in a double blind placebo-controlled study: effects on menopause symptoms and bone markers. *Maturitas* 2003; **44 (suppl 1)**: S67–77.

8 Phytoestrogens and bone health

Aedin Cassidy

Introduction

The option of using dietary phytoestrogens for the prevention of osteoporosis is gaining momentum. Much of the evidence for a role in bone health, however, relates to animal data, as most of the available human studies are of short duration and have used either bone biomarkers or bone mineral density as endpoint measures. The potential ability of these compounds to reduce bone loss in postmenopausal women in randomized long-term trials has not been investigated, and an assessment of their effect on fracture rates will be critical in the future.

The lower reported rates of hip fracture in Asian populations compared with western populations has stimulated significant interest in the potential role of dietary phytoestrogens (present mainly in soya) as protective agents for bone health.

Dietary sources of phytoestrogens

The main class of dietary phytoestrogens that has received attention is the isoflavones. Their occurrence in foods is limited largely to soybeans and a few other legumes. Although isoflavones have weak oestrogenic activity, some foods and dietary supplements contain comparatively high amounts of these compounds, so these compounds have the potential to exert biological effects *in vivo*. Daily dietary intake of isoflavones in western populations is typically negligible (<1 mg/day). The rapidly changing eating trends in Japan or China now make it difficult to determine accurately the intake of isoflavones in these countries, where soy is traditionally consumed as a staple. Recent estimates indicate intakes of 20–50 mg/day, but this may vary between urban and rural areas and with other lifestyle factors.

Although all soybean derived protein extracts and foods available for human consumption contain significant levels of isoflavones, large variability is seen in the concentration and profile among these products and depends on species, geographical and environmental conditions and the extent of industrial processing.

The highest levels of isoflavones are found in soy flours and soy protein concentrates; tofu and soymilks also contain significant amounts, although concentrations vary considerably between type and brand. In recent years, numerous extracts of soy or other sources of isoflavones (such as red clover) have been produced commercially as supplements, but recent data suggest that quality assurance is a significant issue with commonly available

47

isoflavone supplements, and, to date, data examining their relative clinical effectiveness are limited.

Mechanisms of action

These bioactive compounds are structurally similar to the mammalian oestrogen oestradiol and thus are viewed as possible selective oestrogen receptor modulators. They also possess other non-oestrogen receptor mediated properties that may contribute to their potential bone sparing properties.

Their cellular actions are determined by many factors, including the relative levels of oestrogen receptors α and β, the range of coactivators and corepressors present in any given cell type, and the nature of the response elements with which the receptors interact with oestrogen-regulated genes. That the resulting effects observed from *in vitro* and *in vivo* experiments are inconsistent is not surprising, as the biological effects vary depending on the phytoestrogen compound studied, the cell line used and the species and tissue under examination. Furthermore there is also significant variation in gastrointestinal metabolism of phytoestrogens.

Any potential beneficial effect of isoflavones on bone tissues could result from increased bone formation by osteoblasts or decreased bone resorption by osteoclasts. Either mechanism could increase bone mass and thus help prevent the development of osteoporosis. Phytoestrogens may act directly on osteoblasts by genomic mechanisms involving activation or inhibition of nuclear oestrogen receptors. Dietary phytoestrogens may help to prevent bone resorption and bone loss by enhancing osteoblastic production of osteoprotegerin, which is an important inhibitor of the terminal differentiation and activation of osteoclasts. Alternatively, a variety of non-genomic mechanisms, including inhibition of tyrosine kinase and inhibition of topoisomerases, have been proposed as the mechanisms of action of phytoestrogens. Genistein acts on osteoblast-like cells by increasing cell proliferation and also protects against oxidative cellular damage of free radicals in these cells. The inhibition of osteoclast activity may also result from a direct action of phytoestrogens, presumably via non-genomic mechanisms, as mammalian osteoclasts lack oestrogen receptors; or from an indirect action mediated by inhibitory cytokines released by osteoblasts in response to the actions of phytoestrogens.

Animal data

To date, much of the evidence for a role of phytoestrogens in bone health has stemmed from animal data, predominantly from studies conducted in rodents and primates. The consensus from these data has shown that phytoestrogens improve the retention of bone mass after ovariectomy. Low doses of genistein (1 mg/day) increased bone retention in oophrectomized lactating rats: similar to the effects observed with conjugated equine oestrogens. High doses of 5 mg/day were less effective. These data thus support the concept that a critical dose is required before any measurable effect on bone mass and density can be observed, and that consumption of high doses of these compounds may be less effective.

Although the consensus of data from rodent studies shows that soy isoflavones are effective at reducing bone loss and increasing bone formation, two studies with ovariectomized cynomolgus monkeys failed to show an effect. In these studies, the positive controls for animals fed conjugated equine oestrogen and oestradiol showed the expected reduction in bone turnover. The lack of effect of isoflavones therefore may vary between species and may well relate to interspecies differences in the metabolic handling of these compounds. Rats rapidly metabolize isoflavones to the most potent precursor equol, and this may account for the biological effects of isoflavones in this species.

Human studies

To date, little data in humans support the potentially protective role of phytoestrogens in relation to bone health. Most of the intervention studies conducted to date are of relatively short duration. Overall, these dietary studies have shown positive effects that may be interpreted as beneficial, but to tease out the precise contribution that phytoestrogens play in the overall endpoints measured is difficult. In particular, to date, insufficient data are available to ascertain the optimal dose of isoflavones needed to exert specific clinical effects.

Several cohort studies suggest that high intake of soy phytoestrogen may be protective for bone mineral density. Habitual intake of high levels of soy products (>50 mg/day isoflavones from soy foods) resulted in a significant increase in bone mineral density compared with the lowest intake group (<35 mg/day), even after adjustment for weight and years since menopause.

Several studies (3–24 months' duration) have examined the effects of phytoestrogen-rich foods on bone mineral density in perimenopausal and postmenopausal women (Table 1). Although the studies used different designs and durations of intervention and varied in the amount of soy foods fed overall, the data are suggestive of a positive effect in the lumbar spine at higher intakes (>60 mg/day).

Some intervention studies also have used biomarkers of bone health as endpoint measures. These studies also vary by design, duration, menopausal status, dose of isoflavones and biomarker measures. Overall, however, these studies suggest lower levels of bone resorption markers with higher soy intake. Only two long-term studies have examined the role of soy products or isoflavone compounds on bone density. In a placebo-controlled trial, intervention with genistein resulted in an increase in bone mineral density at the femoral neck, Ward's triangle and lumbar spine, and

protective changes were seen in urinary and serum bone biomarkers. In a two-year intervention study, the results suggested that long-term consumption of 100 mg/day isoflavones (fed as two glasses of soy milk) prevented the expected decrease in bone mineral density of the lumbar spine.

Ipriflavone

The biological activity of the naturally occurring phytoestrogens led to research and development of synthetic derivatives for pharmacological use. The best known example is the isoflavone derivative ipriflavone, whose chemical structure is similar to the isoflavone precursor daidzein. Until recently, ipriflavone was used in several countries as an alternative to hormone replacement therapy for preventing bone loss, but safety and efficacy data were conflicting. The recent publication of a randomized controlled trial, however, showed that it did not prevent bone loss or affect biochemical markers of bone metabolism and, in addition, ipriflavone induced lymphocytopaenia in a significant number of patients.

Safety issues

A range of phytoestrogen-enriched food products and supplements are available but, to date, most of these products are supported by limited clinical evidence of effectiveness and safety. Such clinical data are critical so that women can be assured that these products are safe for long-term consumption, are effective and pose no greater risk then HRT.

Other health effects

The international variation in many other diseases, including cardiovascular disease, menopausal symptoms and breast cancer, has stimulated interest in the role of isoflavones in the diet as potentially protective components.

Table 1
Human intervention studies on phytoestrogens and bone health.

Study	Design	Number of participants	Duration (months)	Source	Isoflavone Dose (mg/day)	Outcome measure
Short term (<6 months' duration)						
Murkies et al (1995)	Parallel arm	58	3	Soybean flour	74	• Decrease urinary hydroxyproline
Dalais et al (1998)	RCT	52	3	Soya foods	53	• BMD (NS)
Scheiber et al (2000)	Open design (no placebo)	42	3	Soybean foods	60	• Increase BMC (5.2%) • Osteocalcin (NS) • Decrease urinary N-telopeptide
Scambia et al (2000)	RCT, crossover	39	1.5	Soy extract	50	• Osteolcalcin (NS)
Wangen et al (2000)	RCT, crossover	17	3	Soy protein isolate	8, 65 and 130	• Bone biomarkers (NS)
Upmalis et al (2000)	RCT, double blind	175	3	Soy isoflavone extract	50	• Osteocalcin (NS) • Urinary N-telopeptide (NS)
Uesugi et al (2002)	RCT, crossover	23	1	Soy isoflavone extract	62	• Decrease urinary deoxypyridinoline
Medium term (≥6 months' duration)						
Potter et al (1998)	RCT, double blind	66	6	Soy protein isolate	90	• Increase lumbar BMD 2.2%
Alekel et al (2000)	RCT, double blind	69	6	Soy protein isolate	4 and 80	• Increase BMC 0.6% (80mg dose) • Decreased lumbar spine bone loss
Clifton-Bligh et al 2001	RCT, double blind	46	6	Red clover	28, 57 and 85	• Decreased lumbar spine bone loss
Hsu et al (2001)		37	6	Isoflavone supplement	300	• Increase BMD (57 & 85 mg doses)
Lydeking-Olsen et al (2002)	RCT	89	2 years	Soymilk	100	• BMD (NS) • Decreased lumbar spine bone loss
Chiechi et al (2002)	RCT	187	6	Soyfoods		• Increase osteoclacin, urinary hydroxyproline (NS) • BMD (NS)
Morabito et al (2002)	RCT	90	1 year	Genistein	54	• Increase BMD • Decrease urinary pyridinoline, deoxypyridinoline • Increase osteocalcin and alkaline phosphatase

RCT = randomized controlled trial; NS = non-significant; BMD = bone mineral density; BMC = bone mineral content

In Asia, where urine and plasma levels of these compounds are high, these conditions are rare. However, to date, clinical studies that have examined the potential of isoflavones to cause physiological effects in humans have been limited to epidemiological studies or to dietary intervention trials, which have examined effects on menopausal symptoms, cardiovascular risk biomarkers and endocrine regulation of the menstrual cycle. Overall, these dietary studies have shown positive effects that may be interpreted as beneficial, but it is difficult to tease out the precise contribution that isoflavones play in the overall endpoint measures. In particular we have insufficient data to ascertain the optimal dose of isoflavone necessary to exert clinical effects and to determine the relative benefits of supplements containing these compounds over soy foods naturally rich in phytoestrogens.

Conclusions

Given the risk–benefit profile of hormone replacement therapy, further research to determine the relative importance of naturally occurring phytoestrogens in women's health will be important in the future. Much of the evidence for a role of phytoestrogens in bone health comes from animal data; however, recent long-term studies in humans suggest that a dose of 100 mg/day from soy foods can prevent the expected loss in bone mineral density in postmenopausal women. Such clinical data are critically important so that women can be confident that these products are safe for long-term consumption and that they pose no greater risk than HRT. Further studies are underway, including a European Union study (Phytos), which should help to further quantify the relative importance of these compounds and define optimal dose for bone-preserving effects.

Further reading

Adlercreutz H, Honjo H, Higashi A, et al. Urinary excretion of lignans and isoflavonoid phytoestrogens in Japanese men and women consuming a traditional Japanese diet. Am J Clin Nutr 1991; 54: 1093–100.

Alexandersen P, Toussaint A, Christiansen C, et al. Ipriflavone in the treatment of postmenopausal osteoporosis. JAMA 2001; 285: 1482–8.

Anderson JJB, Garner SC. Phytoestrogens and bone. Clin Endocrinol Metab 1998; 12: 543–57.

Anderson JJ, Ambrose WW, Garner SC. Biphasic effect of genistein on bone tissue in the ovariectomized, lactating rat model. PSEBM 1998; 217: 345–50.

Branca F. Dietary phyto-oestrogens and bone health. Proc Nut Soc 2003; 62: 877–87.

Cassidy A. Phytoestrogens and bone health. J Br Menopause Soc 2003; 9: 17–21.

Lee YS, Chen XW, Anderson JJB. Physiological concentrations of genistein stimulate the proliferation and protect against free radical induced oxidative damage of MC3T3-E1 osteoblast-like cells. Nutr Res 2001; 21: 1287–98.

Lees C-J, Ginn T-A. Soy isolate diet does not prevent increased cortical bone turnover in ovariectomized macaques. Calcif Tissue Intl 1998; 62: 557–8.

Montano MM, Katzenellenbogen BS. The quinone reductase gene: a unique estrogen receptor-regulated gene that is activated by antioestrogens. PNAS USA 1997; 94: 2581–6.

Rowland IR, Wiseman H, Sanders TA, et al. Interindividual variation in metabolism of soy isoflavones and lignans: influence of habitual diet on equol production by the gut microflora. Nutr Cancer 2000; 36(1): 27–32.

Setchell KDR, Cassidy A. Dietary isoflavones: biological effects and relevance to human health. J Nutr 1999; 129: 758S–767S.

Setchell, KDR, Brown, NM, Desai P, et al. Bioavailability of pure isoflavones in healthy humans and analysis of commercial soy isoflavone supplements. J Nutr 2001; 131 (4 suppl): 1362S–175S.

Somekawa Y, Chiguchi M, Ishibashi T, et al. Soy intake related to menopausal symptoms, serum lipids and bone mineral density in postmenopausal Japanese women. Obstet Gynecol 2001; 97: 109–15.

Tobias JH, Cook DG, Chambers TJ, Datzell N. A comparison of bone mineral density between Caucasian, Asian and Afro-Caribbean women. Clin Sci 1994; 87: 587–9.

Valtuena S, Cahsman K, Robins SP, et al. Investigating the role of natural phyto-oestrogens on bone health in postmenopausal women. Br J Nutr 2003; 89: S87–99.

9

Homeopathy and the menopause

Elizabeth A Thompson

Introduction

Homeopathy is one of a number of complementary therapies that women actively seek for their menopausal symptoms, and such symptoms are a common cause of referral to the five National Health Service homeopathic hospitals in the UK. This chapter describes the rationale behind homeopathic prescribing and its use in the menopause. Research findings will be discussed with regard to scientific and clinical evidence of a biological action for homeopathic dilutions, along with data that suggest that the homeopathic approach can offer relevant symptom control for menopausal women and women with breast cancer and symptoms of oestrogen withdrawal.

What is homeopathy?

The homeopathic approach does not just concern a remedy but has a patient led consultation that is symptom or problem orientated. During the consultation, each prescription is individualized to reflect the diversity of human nature. A 'local' rather than individualized prescription also may be recommended, which reflects mainly physical symptoms. For example, amyl nitrosum is a remedy that has found to be useful in the menopause. The symptom picture of this remedy is described in one homeopathic materia medica as 'producing flushings of face,

heat, and throbbing in the head...and other discomforts at climacteric'. The nature of these symptom pictures will be described more fully below.

Background to homeopathy

Samuel Hahnemann (1755–1843), a German physician and scientist, first began to uncover the central tenets of homoeopathic philosophy. Where Descartes had reduced the human body to a machine, Hahnemann believed in the vital force – that which animates and regulates the human form and directs growth, healing and repair. He postulated that the homoeopathic remedy acted through the vital force to stimulate a healing or self-regulating response.

Hahnemann began to draw out patterns of symptoms in relation to homoeopathic medicines, in a process called a 'proving'. The first proving (*prüfung* means a trial of a substance) used chinchona, the bark of the Peruvian yew, which is known for its beneficial action in malaria and from which quinine is derived. When given to a healthy person, Hahnemann found that a pattern of symptoms developed similar to those found in a patient with malaria. He went on to build up a catalogue of these symptom pictures with a variety of substances including *Belladonna* (deadly nightshade) and *Arsenic*. Symptom pictures particular to a medicine could be matched to the symptoms in the ill person. Once he had discovered that medicines given in this way could be curative in acute diseases, he stated the fundamental law of similars: 'let like be treated with like'. Some psychotherapeutic techniques might be said to share this homoeopathic approach: focusing, clarifying and reflecting back the same story with the hope of stimulating a healing response. Examples of conventional drugs that create the symptoms they are used to treat and thus illustrate the homeopathic principle include:

- amphetamine, which induces hyperactivity and is used in hyperactivity disorder
- aspirin, which is used in fever and has hyperthermia as a side-effect
- chemotherapy, which both treats and causes malignancy.

Provings are undertaken to this present day, as infinite symptom pictures can be ascertained from plant, mineral and animal sources.

Hahnemann pursued the minimum dose – the smallest amount of a substance that could be given to avoid side-effects and yet would still bring about a healing response. Much to his surprise, the curative action of certain preparations seemed to be stronger at some of the lower doses, particularly when shaken vigorously (a process known as succussion), than at higher doses.

Scientific research

Hahnemann had chanced on the observation that very low doses of a substance seemed to stimulate a healing response. Modern pharmacology has traditionally taught that very low concentrations of medicines have little or no effect on living mechanisms. As early as the 1940s in the fields of radiation and toxicology research, certain toxins in high doses were observed to inhibit metabolism and ultimately cause death but at low doses they produced a stimulatory effect. As evidence

accumulated, the phenomenon became known as hormesis, which refers to a biphasic dose–response relationship, in which higher doses cause an inhibitory effect and lower doses a stimulatory effect.

Homeopathy is sometimes confused with herbal medicines, although the preparation of homeopathic remedies is different. After initial trituration of the substance, the mixture is taken through a process of dilution and succussion known as potentization. Succussion is defined as serial agitation of a solution. It is counterintuitive to imagine that a substance can become more potent at the same time as it is rendered more dilute. Interesting research from Korea, however, found that when certain substances are diluted in water, the molecules clump together instead of getting further apart as common sense would suggest. As the dilution increases, the clusters grow large enough to interact with biological tissues. It is possible that the process of succussion encourages the aggregates to get larger and this enhances the biological effect.

These homeopathic dilutions have been referred to as ultramolecular dilutions. One theory put forward for ultramolecular dilutions is the possibility that water may carry information, just like ferrous oxide can be a carrier for sound. Beneveniste, who described this idea, supported research within his department, which showed a biological action of an ultramolecular dilution of anti-immunoglobulin E (IgE). His department subsequently was closed down, but 13 years later, similar research was reported by Belon *et al* in a multicentre European study. The research teams found that high dilutions of histamine do inhibit anti-IgE-induced basophil degranulation. The lead researcher for this study has been 'forced to suspend my disbelief and seek for a rational explanation for these findings'.

Clinical research

In a meta-analysis of over 100 trials with homeopathy, over 77% were positive, and the independent authors suggested further research was warranted. The results of a more recent meta-analysis of placebo-controlled trials of homeopathy were not compatible with the hypothesis that the clinical effects of homeopathy are completely due to the placebo effect.

Pilot and observational study data for homeopathy and the menopause

A body of observational data was collected from homeopathic hospitals around the UK with an outcome score based on a seven-point scale. The outcome is rated by the patient in consultation with the doctor and +2 or +3 on these scores are regarded as treatment successes, with changes large enough to improve quality of life or reflect a major improvement in symptoms. An average of 61% of women who continued to attend outpatients for more than one follow-up visit rated an outcome of +2 or +3 on this score for their menopausal symptoms across three centres. This is compared with 70% of attendees to the Royal London Homeopathic Hospital Women's Clinic who experienced a definite improvement in symptoms, although no mention of the outcome score used to make these assessments is made.

A recent publication reported an uncontrolled, pilot outcome study of 31 women with hot flushes who attended a homeopathic outpatient centre. For all patients, the initial and follow up assessments included a review of the frequency and severity of hot flushes. Patients also completed their own self-assessment rating after follow-up consultations. The results indicate useful symptomatic benefit for all three groups (women with hot flushes without breast cancer, women with hot flushes and a history of breast cancer and women with hot flushes and breast cancer patients who were using tamoxifen).

Randomized controlled trials for homeopathy and the menopause

Two randomized studies have evaluated the use of homeopathy for menopausal symptoms in the non-cancer setting. Both found an improvement with homeopathy, but the number of patients was small and no statistically significant differences were found when compared with placebo.

Clinical research for women with breast cancer and symptoms of oestrogen withdrawal

In an observational study that investigated the homeopathic approach to symptom control, women with breast cancer and menopausal symptoms were the most frequent attendees to the designated cancer clinic. Symptom scores in general improved significantly over the study period (p value = 0.001), and evaluable data on 26 women with hot flushes showed significant improvements (p value = 0.046). To look at this sample more closely, women referred with breast cancer and menopausal symptoms continued to be recruited at the end of the prospective observational study until data on 45 women could be analysed.

Of these 45 women, 55% of whom were taking tamoxifen, the most common presenting symptoms were hot flushes (n value = 38), mood disturbance (n value = 23), joint pains (n value = 12) and fatigue (n value = 16). Other symptoms included sleeplessness, lowered libido, weight gain, cystitis, vaginal dryness and skin eruptions. Forty (89%) women completed the study. Significant improvements in mean symptom scores were seen over the study period and for the primary endpoint: effect on daily living scores. Symptoms other than hot flushes, such as fatigue and mood disturbance, were helped significantly. Quality of life improved significantly and satisfaction with the homeopathic approach was high.

Randomized placebo-controlled trials for women with breast cancer and symptoms of oestrogen withdrawal

One randomized controlled trial has been completed and another is underway in the US.

Side-effects

Side-effects do occur with homeopathic remedies. As discussed above, if the method of developing symptom pictures is to give the medicine to healthy volunteers, then giving repeated doses could lead to symptoms of the remedy appearing over time. These are called new or proving symptoms; they are fairly unusual as in most cases just a few doses of the medicine are given. The more common side-effect is an aggravation of symptoms, which usually occurs within 10 days of taking the medicine and is relatively short lived. If a woman has an aggravation of her menopausal symptoms while taking repeated doses of the medicine, it is important to recommend that she stop the remedy and watch and wait. If the medicine is a good match for her symptoms, the symptoms should gradually settle and show an overall improvement from baseline. In one recent study of 116 patients who attended an outpatient unit, 13 (9%) women regarded the side-effects of medication as adverse; however, most tolerated medicines very well. This figure compares with a systematic review of homeopathic side-effects in which the mean incidence was 9.4% in randomized controlled trials.

Conclusion

Homeopathy has been used clinically for more than 150 years. Basic science suggests that a biological response to ultramolecular dilutions exists, although the mechanism of this response is unclear. Data from case histories and observational data suggest that the homeopathic approach can offer a clinically relevant choice for women with menopausal symptoms and for women with breast cancer and menopausal symptoms whether or not they are taking tamoxifen. Most of this data comes from uncontrolled trials, and more research is clearly needed. The results of two randomized controlled clinical trials will be published in the near future. In the meantime, the homeopathic approach seems to be safe, with minimal side-effects, is inexpensive and gives high levels of satisfaction.

Further reading

Belon P, Cumps J, Ennis M, et al. Inhibition of human basophil degranulation by successive histamine dilutions: results of a European multi-centre trial. Inflamm Res 1999; **48 (suppl 1)**: S17–18.

Calabrese EJ, Baldwin LA. Defining hormesis. Hum Exp Toxicol 2002; **21**: 91–7.

Clover A. Patient benefit survey: Tunbridge Wells Homoeopathic Hospital. Br Homeopath J 2000; **89**: 68–72.

Clover A. Homeopathic treatment of hot flushes: a pilot study. Homeopathy 2002; **91**: 75–9.

Dantas F, Rampes H. Do homeopathic medicines provoke adverse effects? A systematic review. Br Homeopath J 2000; **89 (suppl 1)**: S35–8.

Davenas E, Beauvais F, Amara J, et al. Human basophil degranulation triggered by very dilute antiserum against IgE. Nature 1988; **333**: 816–18.

Katz T. Homoeopathic treatment during the menopause. Complement Ther Nurs Midwifery 1997; **3**: 46–50.

Kleijnen J, Knipschild P, ter Riet G. Clinical trials of homoeopathy. BMJ 1991; **302**: 316–23.

Linde K, Clausius N, Ramirez G, et al. Are the clinical effects of homeopathy placebo effects? A meta-analysis of placebo-controlled trials. Lancet 1997; **350**: 834–43.

Richardson WR. Patient benefit survey: Liverpool Regional Department of Homoeopathic Medicine. Br Homeopath J 2001; **90**: 158–62.

Samal S, Geckeler KE. Unexpected solute aggregation in water on dilution. Chem Commun (Camb) 2001; **21**: 2224–5.

Thompson EA, Reilly D. The homeopathic approach to the treatment of symptoms of oestrogen withdrawal in breast cancer patients. A prospective observational study. Homeopathy 2003; **92**: 131–4.

10 Dehydroepiandrosterone

Joy Hinson and Peter Raven

Introduction

Public interest in dehydroepiandrosterone (DHEA) has increased phenomenally over recent years, as the rumours of its antiageing properties have spread. Unfortunately, these rumours are not backed up by good scientific evidence. Despite this, many people have chosen to self-medicate with DHEA and therefore are mostly outside medical supervision. In some countries, notably the USA, DHEA is widely available over the counter because it is classified as a food supplement. In the UK, DHEA generally is not available at chemists or on prescription, but many websites offer it for sale. These sites often contain greatly exaggerated claims about the possible benefits of taking DHEA. This chapter will explain how DHEA has come to be seen as a desirable drug to take and examine the evidence for its therapeutic value in the menopause.

What is DHEA?

Dehydroepiandrosterone (also known as prasterone) is one of the many steroid hormones produced by the adrenal gland (Figure 1). It is mostly produced in a sulphated form (DHEAS) which may be converted to DHEA in many tissues of the body. The regulation of DHEA(S) secretion by the adrenal gland is not well understood, but it is clear that the actions of

adrenocorticotrophin (ACTH), the major adrenal stimulant, do not fully account for the secretion pattern of DHEA. There is also uncertainty as to whether DHEA is active itself (it has been shown to act as both a weak androgen and oestrogen), or whether it first has to be converted in the body into more active hormones, which may be either androgens or oestrogens. It is possible that the second of these mechanisms is more relevant in postmenopausal women as the conversion of DHEA to oestrogens is known to increase with age.

Why consider taking DHEA?

Two aspects of the biology of DHEA have led some practitioners to recommend its therapeutic use – in the menopause and in other conditions. First, blood concentrations of DHEA are at their peak in early adulthood. From the age of around 30 years, concentrations of DHEA begin to decline, until by the age of 80 years they are barely 10% of peak levels (Figure 2). This phenomenon of an age-related decline in DHEA has been termed 'adrenopause'. Second, in patients with almost all chronic medical conditions – from diabetes mellitus to rheumatoid arthritis and coronary heart disease – DHEA levels are significantly lower than in healthy people of the same age. It is, of course, not clear from these studies whether a low circulating DHEA is the cause of illness or a result of it.

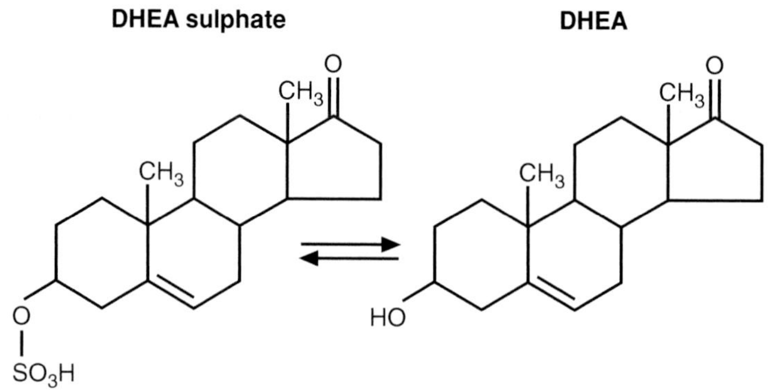

DHEA sulphate   **DHEA**

Figure 1
Structure of DHEA and its sulphated form DHEAS.

From these observations, however, some have concluded that DHEA is a hormone of youth and 'wellness' and that various disorders, even the effects of ageing itself, may be ameliorated by DHEA therapy.

Possible benefits of taking DHEA

One of the major problems in evaluating the possible use of DHEA in the menopause, as in other conditions, is the lack of large, adequately controlled clinical trials. Even where such trials have been conducted, variations in the dosage, route of administration and duration of treatment make the results difficult to compare. In particular, long-term studies are lacking. Many studies, however, using cells *in vitro* and in animals have suggested that the beneficial effects of DHEA may be very wide ranging. In general, the hope generated by these studies has not been sustained by the results of clinical trials, in which the effects of DHEA seem to be small and often not significant.

Acute menopausal symptoms

Vasomotor symptoms
It is worth noting that no suggestions have been made that DHEA may have a role in treating the acute vasomotor symptoms of the menopause.

Sexual dysfunction
Dehydroepiandrosterone has been shown to increase libido. This effect presumably reflects the weak androgenic actions of DHEA. Vaginal atrophy and dryness are components of menopausal sexual dysfunction, and some evidence shows that DHEA may have a beneficial effect when applied topically as a cream rubbed into the thighs. This effect was achieved without any adverse effects on the endometrium in a 12-month study, but the study was open label in a small group of women, and the result has yet to be repeated.

Mood
Perhaps the most consistently reported beneficial effect of DHEA administration is

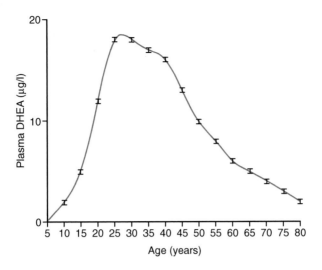

Figure 2
Age related decline in concentrations of dehydroepiandrosterone.

general improvement in mood and increased wellbeing. This effect has been reported in different groups, including people with adrenal insufficiency and those who are taking long-term treatment for chronic inflammatory disease. Although the effects of DHEA on mood seem to be universal and more pronounced in women, studies to date have not specifically addressed the effect on mood disorder in perimenopausal women.

Long-term effects of the menopause

Dehydroepiandrosterone has been proposed to have a role in the prevention of some of the long-term consequences of the menopause. Epidemiological studies have suggested that high endogenous concentrations of DHEA may offer some protection against loss of bone mass and help maintain immune function. Animal studies suggest that treatment with DHEA can bring about beneficial changes in body composition and circulating lipids. In general, however, administration of DHEA to people has

not been found to have any major effects in these areas.

Osteoporosis
Bone mineral density (BMD) has been shown to correlate positively with plasma concentrations of endogenous DHEA in older women, so it is proposed that high circulating DHEA may have a protective effect on bone. Unfortunately, administration of DHEA does not seem to mimic the effects of high concentrations of the endogenous hormone, as giving DHEA to postmenopausal women had only a small effect on bone mineral density of the hip and spine.

Cardiovascular disease
To date, no study has been conducted to determine whether administration of DHEA can reduce the incidence of cardiovascular disease. Several studies, however, have looked at the effects of DHEA administration on various risk factors. There is no good evidence that DHEA has beneficial effects on body mass composition, circulating fatty acids or insulin resistance.

Other potential beneficial effects

Attempts to use DHEA as an immune adjuvant to boost responses to influenza vaccine, for example, have not produced an increase in the number of responders. Among those people who do respond to the vaccine, however, DHEA seems to increase the response. In patients with autoimmune diseases, such as systemic lupus erythematosus, evidence shows that administration of DHEA reduces the severity of the disease, with fewer acute flare-ups.

Adverse effects

In general, DHEA seems to be well tolerated. Most of the adverse effects reported relate to androgenic effects: increased sebaceous secretion, sweating and acne. These effects have been reported even at physiological replacement doses. The adverse effects of DHEA, however, are likely to be significantly underreported, as many people take DHEA outside of medical supervision.

Of most concern, however, is the possibility that DHEA may increase the risk of developing certain cancers. Various *in vitro* and animal studies have suggested that DHEA may promote the growth of breast cancer cells. In addition, a prospective study showed that postmenopausal women with high circulating concentrations of DHEA are at higher risk of developing breast cancer. It should be noted that this subject is at present highly controversial, and strong arguments have been put forward that DHEA is protective against breast cancer and even inhibits tumour progression. Further studies will be needed before this issue can be resolved.

Conclusion

Few definite conclusions can be made about the value of DHEA therapy given our present state of knowledge. DHEA alone, however, is unlikely to be an effective treatment for all the symptoms of the menopause.

Dehydroepiandrosterone has been suggested to have beneficial effects on some symptoms, but the lack of large, placebo-controlled trials makes the possible benefits of DHEA difficult to evaluate. In this respect, the menopause is similar to the other conditions for which treatment with DHEA has been proposed. Uncertainty remains about the beneficial effects of taking DHEA and the possible long-term side-effects. Further studies are urgently needed to clarify these issues.

Further reading

Casson PR, Andersen RN, Herrod HG, et al. Oral dehydroepiandrosterone in physiologic doses modulates immune function in postmenopausal women. Am J Obstet Gynecol 1993; **169**: 1536–9.

Casson PR, Santoro N, Elkind-Hirsch K, et al. Postmenopausal dehydroepiandrosterone administration increases free insulin-like growth factor-1 and decreases high-density lipoprotein: a six month trial. Reproductive Endocrinology 1998; **70**: 107–10.

Danenberg HD, Ben-Yehuda A, Zakay-Rones Z, et al. Dehydroepiandrosterone treatment is not beneficial to the immune response to influenza in elderly subjects. J Clin Endocrinol Metab 1997; **82**: 2911–4.

Greendale GA, Edelstein S, Barrett-Connor E. Endogenous sex steroids and bone mineral density in older women and men: the Rancho-Bernado study. J Bone Miner Res 1997; **12**: 1833–43.

Harper AJ, Buster JE, Casson PR. Changes in adrenocortical function with aging and therapeutic implications. Semin Reprod Endocrinol 1999; **17**: 327–38.

Hinson JP, Raven PW. DHEA deficiency syndrome: a new term for old age? J Endocrinol 1999; **163**: 1–5.

Labrie F, Diamond P, Cusan L, et al. Effect of 12-month dehydroepiandrosterone replacement therapy on bone, vagina and endometrium in postmenopausal women. J Clin Endocrinol Metab 1997; **82**: 3498–505.

Labrie F, Luu-The V, Labrie C, et al. Endocrine and Intracrine sources of androgens in women: inhibition of breast cancer and other roles of androgens and their precursor dehydroepiandrosterone. Endocrine Rev 2003; **24**: 152–82.

Lasco A, Frisina N, Morabito N, et al. Metabolic effects of dehydroepiandrosterone replacement therapy in postmenopausal women. Eur J Endocrinol 2001; **145**: 457–61.

Marcelli C. Can DHEA be used to prevent bone loss and osteoporosis? Joint Bone Spine 2003; **70**: 1–2.

Morales AJ, Nolan JJ, Nelson JC, Yen SSC. Effects of replacement dose of dehydroepiandrosterone in men and women of advancing age. J Clin Endocrinol Metab 1994; **78**: 1360–7.

Raven PW, Hinson JP. DHEA and the menopause: a new approach to HRT? *J Br Menopause Soc* 2001; **7**: 175–80.

Stoll BA. Dietary supplements of dehydroepiandrosterone in relation to breast cancer risk. *Eur J Clin Nutrition* 1999; **53**: 771–5.

Svec F, Porter JR. The actions of exogenous dehydroepiandrosterone in experimental animals and humans. *Soc Exp Biol Med* 1998; **218**: 174–91.

11 Transdermal progesterone creams

Margaret Rees

Introduction

Progesterone creams are advocated for the treatment of menopausal symptoms and skeletal protection. Progesterone is one of a number of hormones produced by the ovary and the placenta. During the menstrual cycle, this steroid has a number of functions, including inhibition of mitotic activity and induction of secretory change in the endometrium.

Although oestrogen is the major steroid administered to control menopausal symptoms and conserve bone mass, progesterone and progestogens have a significant part to play in regimens for women whose uterus is intact. They are added to reduce the risk of endometrial hyperplasia and cancer that would occur with oestrogen alone. Progesterone is produced commercially by multiple enzymatic conversion of precursors, such as diosgenin found in wild yam. Given orally, however, progesterone is inactivated by enzymatic degradation in the gut and liver. This has led to the production of more stable compounds called progestogens, such as norethisterone and levonorgestrel, which also have a progestogenic effect on the endometrium. They can be given orally, some are given transdermally, and levonorgestrel is delivered by an intrauterine device. These compounds can be manufactured from plant sources, such as soya beans and yams. Women may experience various side-effects from progestogens, however, which has led to the search for a more 'natural' alternative.

Transdermal progesterone preparations

Progesterone has been prepared in gels and creams for a number of years. One licensed gel is available in Europe; however, it is indicated for local use on the breast but not for systemic therapy. A vaginal gel for endometrial protection has been studied, but availability is limited. The various transdermal preparations for systemic use usually contain micronized progesterone in concentrations ranging from 0.17 mg/g to 64.0 mg/g, with most products containing about 30.0 mg/g in a cream. Some of the major supporters of transdermal progesterone cream are based in the USA. No good evidence, however, shows that transdermal progesterone creams can achieve biologically active levels in plasma or are capable of protecting the endometrium from hyperplasia or conserving bone mass.

Endometrial effects

To avoid the side-effects of progestogens, women who take oestrogens may use transdermal progesterone creams for endometrial protection. No good consistent evidence, however, shows that transdermal progesterone creams prevent mitotic activity or induce secretory change in an oestrogen-primed endometrium. Some have suggested that salivary progesterone levels are reliable for monitoring absorption of transdermal creams, but this method has been questioned. Measurement of plasma in short-term studies shows some small and variable increases in plasma levels. For example, Burry et al used a commercially available 30 mg/g micronized progesterone cream in six women and showed that twice daily applications of 1 g increased plasma circulating levels to 1.5–3.5 ng/ml after 15 days of use. Similar findings were obtained by Carey et al with 40 mg/day for 42 days.

These levels, however, are considered insufficient to prevent mitotic activity or induce a secretory effect on the endometrium. Studies are limited and of short duration (28 days). For example, Wren et al (2000) found no secretory changes in the endometrium. They studied 27 postmenopausal women treated with continuous transdermal oestrogen (28 day cycle) and a cream containing 16, 32 or 64 mg progesterone administered daily in a sequential regimen (days 15–28 of the cycle). Leonetti et al (2003), however, used a different cream formulation in 32 women and found that progesterone reduced endometrial proliferation scores. Women were given 0.625 mg of conjugated equine oestrogens and twice daily transdermal application of 0%, 1.5% or 4.0% progesterone cream. The cream's progesterone concentration was based on the patient's weight. Clearly, large, long-term studies are needed.

Menopausal symptoms

Progesterone cream has been promoted for a variety of menopausal symptoms, including hot flushes and moods swings, but results are conflicting. Leonetti et al, in one clinical study of women using a 20 mg/day application of progesterone cream, found no significant effect of progesterone on depression. Vasomotor symptoms, however, were significantly improved by the use of transdermal progesterone. This last observation should be viewed with caution: major differences were present between the two groups at entry, and the women who received a placebo cream for one year had reductions in hot flushes of only 19% (the usual improvement after placebo use over such a period has been noted as 40–70%). Wren et al (2003) undertook a parallel, double-blind, randomized, placebo-controlled trial to compare the effect of a transdermal cream containing progesterone (32 mg daily) with a placebo cream. They were evaluated using the Greene climacteric scale and the menopause quality of life questionnaire, as well as by blood analysis for lipids and bone markers, over a period of 12 weeks. No detectable change in vasomotor symptoms, mood characteristics or sexual feelings was found.

Conservation of bone mass

Progesterone creams have been suggested to conserve bone mass and reduce the risk of osteoporosis; however, no data at present support this claim. Leonetti et al (1999) found no gain in bone mineral density with a 20 mg cream, and Wren et al (2003) found no alteration in bone markers with a 32 mg cream.

Cardiovascular system

The cessation of the oestrogen and progestogens arm of the Women's Health Initiative in 2002 focused again on the cardiovascular effects of various progestogens. Data with transdermal progesterone creams are limited, and no changes in blood lipids have been found. No data on myocardial infarction and stroke, which are arguably the most important endpoints, are available.

Transdermal wild yam cream

Wild yam cream also is popular, but no evidence shows any effect on menopausal

Lifestyle

Role of diet

Brigid McKevith

Introduction

For women who do not want to or cannot use hormone replacement therapy, considerable consideration should be given to the role of diet. The risks of cardiovascular disease, osteoporosis and some cancers (as well as some other health problems) increase as women age. Specific attention should be given to reducing risk factors associated with these conditions, and diet has a key role to play within this risk reduction.

Caloric intake

In the UK, 20% of the adult population are obese [with a body mass index (BMI) over 30 m/kg^2]. As people age, the lean body mass (LBM) declines, mainly as a result of a decrease in skeletal muscle. This decrease in LBM can be minimized if physical activity is maintained or increased. The reduction in LBM seen with age is accompanied by an increase in body fat, specifically in the abdominal area. Energy expenditure decreases with ageing because of a decrease in the basal metabolic rate. As people age, they often become more sedentary, which also decreases energy expenditure. That many people carry excess weight, mainly as fat, as they get older is therefore not surprising.

Obesity is the major risk factor for chronic, life threatening diseases and also is associated with many other health complications (Table 1).

Table 1
Relative risk of health problems associated with obesity. (WHO, 2000)

Greatly increased (relative risk much greater than 3)	Moderately increased (relative risk 2–3)	Slightly increased (relative risk 1–2)
• Type 2 diabetes • Gallbladder disease • Dyslipidaemia • Insulin resistance • Breathlessness	• Coronary heart disease • Hypertension • Osteoarthritis (knee) • Hyperuricaemia and gout	• Cancer (breast cancer in postmenopausal women, endometrial cancer, colon cancer) • Reproductive hormone abnormalities • Polycystic ovary syndrome; impaired fertility • Low back pain • Increased risk of anaesthesia complications • Fetal defects associated with maternal obesity

Some studies have found menopause to be associated with an increase in central body fatness and this may be independent of the ageing process described above.

All women thus should aim to maintain a healthy body weight (BMI 18.50–24.99 m/kg^2). For those who are overweight or obese, weight loss can improve physical health, as well as providing other benefits. In general, energy input must not exceed output, so the total number of calories eaten may have to be controlled. Although older people have reduced energy needs, foods need to be energy dense and to contain the appropriate range of macronutrients (carbohydrate, protein and fat) and micronutrients (vitamins and minerals). Carbohydrate and fat recommendations for healthy older people are the same as for healthy younger adults, but slightly higher amounts of protein may be beneficial for healthy older people (0.9–1.1 g/kg/day).

A sensible weight loss is about 1–2 pounds (about 0.5–1.0 kg) a week. For many people, this means reducing their energy intake by about 1000 kilocalories/day, but this will depend on how much weight loss is needed. Of the three main constituents in food, fat is the most concentrated source of energy, so decreasing consumption of foods that are high in fat can help reduce energy intake. Any dietary plan aimed at weight reduction should be based on the Balance of Good Health (Figure 1).

Fat

Cardiovascular disease (CVD) is the most common cause of morbidity and mortality among women. Several studies have found that menopause is accompanied with increases in total cholesterol and low-density lipoprotein cholesterol. Diet has a major role to play in the

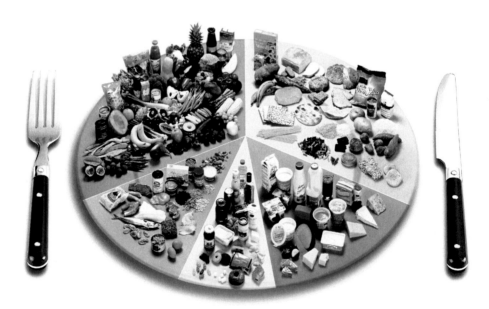

Figure 1
Balance of Good Health. Copyright: British Nutrition Foundation.

prevention of CVD, and epidemiological studies have shown that diets low in saturated fat and high in fruits, vegetables, whole grains and fibre are associated with a decreased risk of coronary heart disease.

In 1994, the UK Committee on Medical Aspects of Food and Nutrition Policy (COMA) made recommendations with regards to total fat and different types of fat (Table 2). Data from the recent National Diet and Nutrition Survey (NDNS) suggest that, although decreasing the intake of total fat has been successful, further work is needed to reduce the amount of saturated fatty acids in the diet (Table 2). For women aged 50–64 years, cheese and butter contributed to the daily intake of saturated fatty acids (10% and 8%, respectively).

Although in the past the main message with regard to fat has been to limit total consumption, omega 3 fatty acids, in particular, may have a special role in the prevention of thrombosis, as well as possible benefits for blood pressure, reducing concentrations of triglycerides and improved insulin sensitivity. Much of the interest in the association between omega 3 fatty acids and cardiovascular disease follows studies with the Greenland Inuits who traditionally have low mortality from coronary heart disease despite a diet rich in fat. Long chain omega 3 fatty acids can be found in oily fish, and current UK recommendations are to consume one portion of oily fish per week.

Calcium and vitamin D

Osteoporosis is an important public health problem that accounts for an estimated 310,000 fractures per year in the UK. A range of factors influence bone health, and menopause marks a time of bone loss in women because of the loss of circulating oestrogen. Adequate nutrition, especially intakes of calcium and vitamin D, and physical activity have pivotal roles in the prevention of osteoporosis. Controlled clinical trials have indicated that among elderly people, adequate calcium and vitamin D intake can reduce bone loss and potentially the risk of fracture.

Calcium is a mineral and is the principal component of bone. The reference nutrient intake (RNI) in the UK for calcium is 700 mg/day, although higher amounts (about 1200 mg/day) are recommended for those diagnosed with osteoporosis. Important dietary sources of calcium include milk and milk products (such as cheese and yoghurt) and cereal and cereal products (these are often fortified with calcium: flour is fortified by legislation in the UK). Calcium can also be obtained from dark green leafy vegetables, tofu, dried fruits, nuts and seeds. Some of these foods, however, contain substances that bind calcium and inhibit its absorption.

Vitamin D is important for bone health, as it is involved in the absorption and excretion of calcium. The RNI for women over the age of 65

Table 2
Recommendations for fat and average intakes in women aged 50–64 years in the UK.

Nutrient	COMA recommendation	Average intake (%)
Total fat	No more than 35% of food energy	34.5
Saturated fatty acids	No more than 11% of food energy	13.3
Trans fatty acids	No more than 2% of food energy	1.2
Polyunsaturated fatty acids		
n-6	Maximum 10% of food energy	5
n-3	0.2 g/day (1.5 g/week)	1.82 g/week

years is 10 µg/day, but for younger women no RNI exists, as vitamin D can be obtained through the action of sunlight on the skin. As this only occurs during the summer months in the UK and other countries at a similar latitude from the equator, and as older skin may have a reduced capacity to produce pre-vitamin D-3, dietary sources such as oily fish, cod liver oil, fortified breakfast cereals and margarine may be important. People who are housebound or live in institutions may be at risk of deficiency. Everyone aged over 65 years thus should be advised to take a vitamin D supplement.

Other factors such as avoiding smoking, limiting alcohol intake, maintaining a healthy body weight, reducing sodium intake and increasing consumption of fruit and vegetables are also important for bone health.

Antioxidants

Antioxidants such as selenium, vitamin E, vitamin C and beta-carotene protect the body from free radical damage. Free radicals are produced during normal metabolism in the body, but they are associated with disease and the ageing process.

Several epidemiological studies have shown that people with high intakes of fruit and vegetables may have a lower risk of chronic disease compared with those with low intakes. The benefits of high intakes of fruits and vegetables are hypothesized to result from their antioxidant content. To date, however, no single antioxidant has been proved to prevent or decrease the risk of chronic disease, so the most practical public health advice is to increase vegetable and fruit consumption.

In the UK, the recommendation is to include at least five portions of fruit and vegetables per day. As the average intake for women aged 50–64 years is still less than this recommendation (3.8 portions), women should be encouraged to eat a wide variety of fruits

and vegetables, as different types provide different profiles of constituents.

Recently, the Food Standards Agency's Expert Committee on Vitamins and Minerals set safe upper limits for some vitamins and minerals, including several of the antioxidant nutrients. Vitamin and mineral supplements may be beneficial to some subgroups of the population, but evidence shows that excessive intakes of some vitamins and minerals can cause harm. For people who take antioxidant supplements, it is important that these safe upper limits are not exceeded:

- beta-carotene 7 mg/day
- vitamin E 727 mg (800 IU)
- selenium 0.3 mg.

For vitamin C, data were insufficient to set a limit.

Conclusion

Women entering the menopause are faced with many challenges. To maintain or achieve a healthy body weight is important, as obesity and being overweight are associated with an increased risk of a variety of health problems. Cardiovascular disease is another risk facing women at this stage of life, and although achieving a fat intake $\leq 35\%$ is important, emphasis should be given to the types of fat in the diet, specifically increasing the intake of omega 3 fatty acids. Adequate intakes of calcium and vitamin D are important for bone health, as are avoiding smoking, limiting alcohol intake and reducing sodium intake. Although much interest surrounds antioxidants, as no single antioxidant has been proved to prevent or reduce the risk of chronic disease, the most practical current public health advice is to increase fruit and vegetable consumption.

Further reading

British Nutrition Foundation. *The report of the British Nutrition Foundation Task Force. Obesity.* Oxford: Blackwell Science, 1999.

Buttriss J. *n-3 Fatty acids and health*. London: British Nutrition Foundation, 1999.

Din JN, Newby DE, Flapan AD. Omega 3 fatty acids and cardiovascular disease – fishing for a natural treatment. *BMJ* 2004; **328**: 30–5.

Goldberg G. *Obesity FLAIR FLOW 4 synthesis report, Health professionals no. 3*. Paris: INRA, 2003.

Henderson L, Gregory J, Irving K, Swan G. *The national diet and nutrition survey: adults aged 19 to 64 years. Energy, protein, carbohydrate, fat and alcohol intake*. London: Stationery Office, 2003.

Henderson L, Gregory J, Swan G. *The national diet and nutrition survey: adults aged 19 to 64 years. Types and quantities of foods consumed*. London: Stationery Office, 2003.

National Heart, Lung, and Blood Institute, Office of Research on Women's Health and Giovanni Lorenzini Medical Science Foundation. *International position paper on women's health and menopause: a comprehensive approach*. Bethesda: National Institutes of Health, 2002.

National Osteoporosis Society. *Primary care strategy for osteoporosis and falls*. Bath: National Osteoporosis Society, 2002.

Phillips F. *Diet and bone health FLAIR FLOW 4 synthesis report. Health professionals no. 5*. Paris: INRA, 2003.

Robinson F. *Nutrition for healthy ageing. FLAIR FLOW 4 synthesis report. Health professionals No. 4*. Paris: INRA, 2003.

World Health Organization. Obesity: preventing and managing the global epidemic. WHO Technical Report Series 894. Geneva: WHO, 2000.

13 Functional foods

Christopher Smejkal

Introduction

Functional foods generally are defined as foods that confer a 'benefit' to the host beyond that of simple nutrition. The current climate is one of increasing interest in such products and the effects of diet on health. Four main types of functional foods show promise in women's health, namely:

- probiotics
- prebiotics
- synbiotics
- nutraceuticals.

Probiotics

Probiotics are defined as 'live microbial feed supplement which beneficially affects the host animal by improving its intestinal balance'. Increasing evidence shows the potential of probiotics in benefiting both gastrointestinal and non-gastrointestinal tract conditions.

Prebiotics

Prebiotics are 'non-digestible food ingredients which selectively stimulate a limited number of bacteria in the colon, to improve host health'. The emphasis of prebiotic research, therefore, is to enhance the indigenous probiotic flora. This includes strategies to develop specific prebiotics for individual probiotic organisms, as well as aiding persistence of prebiotic effects throughout the gastrointestinal tract.

Synbiotics

Synbiotics contain complementary probiotic and prebiotic ingredients that interact to provide a synergistic effect towards the maintenance of a desirable microbial population in the intestinal microbiota. This is a developing area of functional foods and to date few clinical studies have been performed on their impact on human health.

Nutraceuticals

Nutraceuticals are natural components of foods (such as isoflavones and phytoestrogens) that may be released during digestion and therefore become bioavailable. Such compounds may have a direct health effect on host and/or indirect health effect via the microflora.

Probiotics in the treatment of gastrointestinal disorders

Increasing evidence shows that ingested probiotics exert a positive effect on prevention and treatment of specific pathological conditions. Currently, the best studied probiotics are the lactic acid bacteria, particularly *Lactobacillus* spp. and *Bifidobacterium* spp. These can be combined with food products (cereals, bioyoghurts, drinks, etc), for which there is currently a large consumer market.

Diarrhoea and infections

One desirable effect of probiotic supplements is antagonistic activity against pathogens. A well characterized probiotic is *Lactobacillus rhamnosus* GG, which has been shown to have substantial beneficial effects, including the prevention of antibiotic-associated and rotavirus diarrhoea, treatment of relapsing *Clostridium difficile* diarrhoea and enhancement of intestinal immunity. More recently, this strain has been shown to rapidly adhere to human colonic mucosae and thus survive passage through the human gastrointestinal tract. Many lactic acid bacteria can also produce bacteriocins, compounds that are bactericidal and/or bacteriolytic against well known pathogens such as *Listeria* spp, *Salmonella* spp, *Escherichia coli* and *Staphylococcus* spp. More recently, strains of *Lactobacillus* spp. isolated in our laboratory exhibited fungistatic effects on *Candida albicans* and bactericidal effects against the foodborne pathogens *E. coli* EPEC and VTEC.

Candida

The yeast *Candida albicans* is thought to be implicated in gut disorders such as irritable bowel syndrome and gastrointestinal problems in autistic children. This yeast usually remains unproblematic and is a commensal organism of the mouth, genital and intestinal tracts of man. Under certain conditions, however, such as low pH, impaired immune responses or when the normal microflora is suppressed by antibiotic therapy, *Candida* undergoes genetic and physiological changes and causes opportunistic candidiasis that infects the vagina (vaginal

thrush) and/or mouth (oral thrush). Women usually develop yeast related disorders much more commonly than men, and premenopausal women often are most susceptible. The main reasons for this are hormonal changes associated with the menstrual cycle, oral contraceptives and pregnancy. In addition, the anatomical characteristics of women make them more susceptible to urinary tract infections and vaginitis. Evidence shows that probiotic bacteria taken prophylactically or postinfection can help reduce candidiasis and treat the symptoms of recurrent thrush.

Irritable bowel syndrome

Irritable bowel syndrome (IBS) is a common disorder that affects 8–22% of the general population. It is characterized by bloating, abdominal pain, flatulence and changes in bowel habits, with no evidence of organic disease. Some patients with IBS have constipation, while others have diarrhoea and some experience both. Irritable bowel syndrome is prevalent in all age groups, especially women, and it may be extremely painful. Generally, many asymptomatic women experience gastrointestinal disturbances at the time of menstruation, and >50% of women with IBS have an increase in perimenstrual gastrointestinal symptoms. Furthermore, bowel dysfunction is more common in postmenopausal women than in premenopausal women (38% *vs* 14%), and the prevalence of IBS type complaints peaks between the ages of 40 and 49 years. The causes of IBS can be very different between patients (Box 1). Commonly reported food triggers include high-fat foods, caffeine, sorbitol, wheat products and alcohol. Food with excessive fat content encourages the release of cholecystokinin, which stimulates the colon, and large intakes of caffeinated drinks such as coffee and tea stimulate bowel action. Furthermore, strong evidence shows that a depletion of beneficial gut bacteria, such as lactobacilli and bifidobacteria, may also be a contributory factor. Probiotics have been shown to have beneficial effects in patients with IBS, especially those with gastrointestinal infections. A number of studies have shown that prevention of *Helicobacter pylori* infection, as well as reduction of *H. pylori* activity, has been demonstrated by several probiotic bacteria including *L. johnsonii, L. acidophilus* and *B. longum*.

The addition of fibre and prebiotics in the diet is important for central aspects of the digestive process, including:

- nutrient absorption
- sterol metabolism
- bacterial fermentation
- stool weight
- release of short chain fatty acids by bacteria.

Short chain fatty acids are of great importance, because they affect the rate of free water absorption from the faeces by the colonic mucosa and thus provide essential nutrients. Clinical trials using prebiotics and probiotics for the treatment of IBS are very self-limiting to date, and further investigative studies are needed greatly.

Prebiotics in calcium absorption

Calcium is an integral part of human health, as it plays a central role in the development and maintenance of bone tissue. Recent research has focused on the colon as a means of achieving better health through the ingestion of prebiotics. That these dietary components enhance the beneficial bacteria in the human colon, thereby improving host health, is well established. Several researchers have suggested that prebiotics also have a potential role in improving mineral bioavailability and absorption in the colon. A number of possible mechanisms have been proposed:

- bacterial metabolites (short chain fatty acids) lower local pH, dissolving calcium–phosphate–magnesium complexes and thus elevating the luminal concentration of ionized calcium and increasing passive calcium absorption
- modification of the electrical charge of calcium by short chain fatty acids through calcium–hydrogen complexes, which facilitates passage through the membrane.

Animal studies

To date, most studies investigating the effects of prebiotics on calcium absorption and bioavailability have used animal models. Increased calcium absorption occurs in rats after administration of lactulose. Furthermore, as well as increasing calcium absorption, fructooligossacharide (FOS) supplementation counteracts the deleterious effects of phytic acid on mineral homeostasis in rats. Additionally, supplementation with a 1:1 mixture of FOS and cellulose increases absorption and retention of calcium in rats. Animal studies clearly show that prebiotics improve calcium absorption and bone mineralization. Distinct anatomical and physiological differences exist between rodents and humans. As such, research is essential to evaluate the role of prebiotics in calcium absorption in humans. To date, such work is limited.

Human studies

Teuri *et al* investigated the short-term effect of 15 g/day inulin supplementation on calcium metabolism in a randomized, two period, crossover study of 15 healthy young women. No significant effect was observed. Van den Heuvel *et al* similarly showed no detrimental effect of prebiotic supplementation on calcium absorption in a randomized, crossover study of healthy male volunteers. In a later study, the same investigators established that oligofructose administration had no effect (positive or negative) on calcium absorption but that true fractional calcium absorption increased. They also examined the effect of lactulose on calcium absorption in 12 postmenopausal women in a double blind, randomized, crossover trial. A linear trend was found between the dose of lactulose and a positive effect on calcium absorption. Such work is promising; however, further studies are needed to understand the effects of prebiotics on calcium absorption and bone mineralization. When the importance of calcium bioavailability early in life (to achieve peak bone mass) and in later life (to preserve bone integrity) is considered, prebiotics may prove extremely important.

Isoflavones as functional foods

Isoflavones are non-nutrient plant compounds belonging to the phytoestrogen class and have a similar structure to mammalian oestrogens, with a phenolic ring and a 4'-hydroxyl group. The oestrogenic potency of isoflavones and their interaction with oestrogen receptors is low compared with mammalian 17β-oestradiol. The potential of phytoestrogens in the management of the menopause particularly is interesting because of the observed lower incidence of vasomotor symptoms and breast cancer in populations with high dietary soy intake (such as those in Japan and China). Four isoflavones are important:

- genistein
- daidzein
- biochanin
- formononetin.

Red clover also is a good source of phytoestrogens. Randomized trials of soy and red clover on hot flushes have produced conflicting results.

Whether the effect of isoflavones is a direct effect or the result of the longitudinal alterations in hormonal characteristics throughout the life of these people is unclear. Regular inclusion of soy protein in the diet has been correlated with prolongation of the menstrual cycle and suppression of midcycle surges of gonadotrophin, luteinizing and follicle stimulating hormones. A small body of evidence suggests phytoestrogens have the potential to minimize bone loss postmenopausally and this is reviewed in Chapter 8. Soy proteins also have been accredited with hypocholesterolaemic effects, eliciting significant reductions in serum concentrations of total cholesterol and LDL cholesterol. A number of randomized clinical trials have reported hypocholesterolaemic effects of probiotics (certain *Lactobacillus* strains, *Streptococcus thermophilus* and *Enterococcus faecium*). Much debate, however, surrounds the ability of probiotics to lower serum concentrations of cholesterol. Such studies often are confounded with differences in dietary fat content of test and control groups. In addition, initial serum concentrations of cholesterol seem to have an important impact on the effects of dietary intervention – be it probiotic administration or inclusion of phytoestrogens.

The role of the human gut microflora in the metabolism of isoflavones has become a significant research interest and is now fairly well documented and confirmed *in vitro, in vivo* and in a number of animal models. The isoflavone daidzein (from soya) is metabolized extensively in the gut by the human gut microflora to the more oestrogenic secondary metabolite equol. Interest in this compound extends from epidemiological observations that in Asia, where soya consumption is high, rates of various diseases tend to be lower compared with in western populations. Evidence suggests that plasma levels of isoflavones often are elevated in such populations; however, only 30% of western populations excrete high levels of equol. Furthermore, metabolism of diadzein can be altered by other dietary components, such as fat and fibre.

Currently, little research has been undertaken to reliably identify gut bacterial species capable of metabolizing isoflavones. Such data are needed to enable suitable dietary strategies to modify the gut microflora towards converting isoflavones to more protective compounds (including equol).

Conclusion

Evidence to date clearly suggests that functional foods have great potential in aiding the management of the menopause. To ensure clinical evidence is obtained for functional food interventions (whether dietary or topical), however, is essential. The increasing interest in functional foods as alternative therapies means that science is now very much focused on proving their efficacy through ongoing clinical trials. Accurate data, from appropriately designed studies, must be sought for all such products. Several studies, however, show an optimistic future for functional foods in the treatment and alleviation of many disorders associated with the menopause, particularly genitourinary tract and gut related problems.

Further reading

Adlercruetz H, Hamalainen E, Gorbach S, et al. Dietary phytoestrogens and the menopause in Japan [letter]. Lancet 1992; 339: 1233.

Bingham M, Gibson G, Gottstein N, et al. Gut metabolism and cardioprotective effects of dietary isoflavones. Curr Topics Nutraceutical Res 2003; 1: 31–48.

Cashman KD. Calcium intake, calcium bioavailability and bone health. Br J Nutr 2002; 87 (suppl 2): S169–77.

Dixon-Woods M, Critchley S. Medical and lay views of irritable bowel syndrome. Fam Pract 2000; 17: 108–13.

Ernst E. Herbalism and the menopause. J Br Menopause Soc 2002; 8: 72–4.

Frank A. Prebiotics stimulate calcium absorption: a review. Michwissenschaft 1998; 53: 427–9.

Gibson GR, Roberfroid MB. Dietary modulation of the human colonic microbiota: introducing the concept of prebiotics. J Nutr 1995; 125: 1401–12.

Marteau PR, Vrese MD, Cellier CJ, Schrezenmeir J. Protection from gastrointestinal diseases with the use of probiotics. Am J Clin Nutr 2001; 73 (2 suppl): 430S–6S.

Okker DJ, Dicks LMT, Silvester M, et al. Characterization of pentocin TV35b, a bacteriocin-like peptide isolated from Lactobacillus pentosus with a fungistatic effect on Candida albicans. J Appl Microbiol 1999; 87: 726–34.

Payne S, Gibson G, Wynne A, et al. In vitro studies on colonization resistance of the human gut microbiota to Candida albicans and the effects of tetracycline and Lactobacillus plantarum LPK. Curr Issues Intest Microbiol 2003; 4: 1–8.

Reid GR, Burton J. Use of Lactobacillus to prevent infection by pathogenic bacteria. Microbes Infect 2002; 4: 319–24.

Rowland IR, Wiseman H, Sanders TA, et al. Interindividual variation in metabolism of soy isoflavones and lignans: influence of habitual diet on equol production by the gut microflora. Nutr Cancer 2000; 36(1): 27–32.

Setchell KDR, Cassidy A. Dietary isoflavones: biological effects and relevance to human health. J Nutr 1999; 129: 758S–67S.

Teuri U, Karkkainen M, Lamberg-Allardt C, et al. Addition of inulin to breakfast does not acutely affect serum ionized calcium and parathyroid hormone concentrations. Ann Nutr Metab 1999; 43: 356–64.

Tice JA, Ettinger B, Ensrud K, et al. Phytoestrogen supplements for the treatment of hot flashes: the Isoflavone Clover Extract (ICE) Study: a randomized controlled trial. JAMA 2003; 290: 207–14.

Triadafilopoulos G, Finlayson M, Grellet C. Bowel dysfunction in postmenopausal women. Women Health 1998; 27: 55–66.

Trinidad PT, Wolever TMS, Thompson LU. Effect of acetate and propionate on calcium absorption from the rectum and distal colon of man. Am J Clin Nutr 1996; 63: 574–8.

Touhy KM, Probert HM, Smejkal CW, Gibson GR. Using probiotics and prebiotics to improve gut health. Drug Discov Today 2003; 8: 692–700.

Van den Heuvel EG, Muys T, et al. Lactulose stimulates calcium absorption in postmenopausal women. J Bone Miner Res 1999; 14: 1211–16.

Van de Weijer PHM, Barentsen R. Isoflavones from red clover (Promensil*) significantly reduce menopausal hot flush symptoms compared with placebo. Maturitas 2002; 42: 187–93.

14 Exercise and physical interventions

Martin K Oehler

Introduction

A large body of research has established that regular physical activity for postmenopausal women reduces the risk of premature death and disability from a variety of health conditions such as osteoporosis, skeletal fractures, coronary heart disease and type 2 diabetes mellitus. Furthermore, evidence also shows that symptoms often associated with the hormonal changes after menopause, such as hot flushes, urinary incontinence, insomnia and depression, also can be alleviated by physical activity (Box 1). Therefore, exercise is an important modality to maintain health in postmenopausal women.

Despite the growing body of evidence for the benefits of exercise, not only at the menopause but at any age, only 38% of women aged over 19 years are estimated to exercise regularly.

Box 1
Beneficial effects of physical exercise.
- Increases metabolism – loss of weight
- Increases bone mineral density (BMD)
- Increases muscular strength and balance
- Increases cardiovascular fitness
- Improves functional capacity
- Improves mobility
- Improves rehabilitation after fracture
- Improves lipid profiles
- Improves insulin sensitivity
- Improves mood
- Improves menopausal vasomotor episodes
- Improves pelvic floor muscle control

The annual number of lives lost through physical inactivity in the USA is estimated to be more than 250,000.

Exercise methods

Recommended exercise methods for every age group can be divided into three general categories:

- endurance exercise (aerobic)
- strength exercise (resistance)
- balance exercises.

Endurance exercise

Cardiovascular ability (or aerobic capacity) can be increased by appropriate endurance exercise, which greatly improves functional ability. Quite often, carrying out simple activities like making beds, dressing or undressing uses 50% of an elderly person's maximal physical capability, so that the exertion beyond a certain level causes a lack of adequate oxygenation. New participants should start gradually, proceeding from moderate to vigorous aerobic exercise. Low intensity aerobic exercise includes slow walking or chair exercises for people who are unable to walk, while moderate exercise consists of fast walking or recreational sports, such as swimming and cycling, as well as some energetic activities around the house – mowing the lawn or scrubbing floors. Examples of vigorous endurance exercises are climbing stairs, hiking and jogging.

Strength training

Strength training increasingly is recognized as playing an important role in women's health at all ages. Women lose 20–40% of their muscle mass with age. Resistance exercises help restore muscle tissue and can protect vulnerable joints, as well as the lower back. Most strength exercises involve lifting or pushing weights against gravity.

Balancing exercises

Balancing exercises often are modified leg and hip strength exercises and can help prevent falls, which are a common reason for hospitalization in the elderly. In recent years, tai chi, a gentle form of ancient Chinese martial arts, has gained acceptance as a programme that is especially beneficial in improving balance in older women.

It is important that women participate in exercises that are enjoyable, easy to integrate into their daily routine and safe with respect to the risk of exercise induced injuries, as well as dangers attributable to the exercising environment. Group activity usually provides safety, social integration and a more structured routine for participants. Society has to recognize that physical activity is a vital component of a healthy lifestyle and is essential for disease prevention after the menopause.

Osteoporosis

Exercise

The role of exercise in preventing osteoporotic fracture is well supported; however, what type, intensity, frequency and duration of activity is most effective is unclear. Several prospective studies on the effects of exercise training on bone mineral density (BMD) in postmenopausal women suggest that increases in BMD mainly occur when the exercise is quite vigorous (high intensity – for example, workouts with weights) and that low intensity exercise (for example, walking) and

moderate intensity exercise (for example, swimming, cycling) are relatively ineffective in slowing the rate of bone mineral loss.

Nevertheless, results are inconsistent, as various reports show beneficial effects of less strenuous activities, such as walking, on maintaining bone and reducing the risk of hip fractures in postmenopausal women. Walking was reported to increase femoral bone density, is a relatively safe and easy activity and is already the most common exercise among older adults. In one study, walking for four hours/week or more was associated with a 41% lower risk of hip fracture when compared to walking for only one hour/week. Standing was also reported to lower the risk of hip fracture. Similar to a weight bearing activity, standing may confer benefits to balance and muscle strength that may translate into improved bone strength and protection against hip fractures.

A Cochrane review assessed the influence on BMD of different exercise regimens two to three times a week over 12 months in menopausal women. Fast walking effectively improved bone density in the spine and the hip, whereas, on available evidence, weightbearing exercises were associated with increases in bone density of the spine but not the hip.

Vigorous exercise and brisk walking, however, are associated with a higher risk of fall-related fractures, especially in the elderly and in those with functional limitations. For older people, these fractures potentially are very serious, as they have a high mortality (up to 33%) and may result in permanent disability, inability to return to previous living arrangements and the need for nursing-home care. An estimated 1.7 million hip fractures occurred worldwide in 1990 and 6.26 million fractures are predicted to occur by 2050.

Hip protectors

The use of padded hip protectors has been advocated as a measure to reduce the impact of a fall and the risk of consequent hip fracture. Various types of hip protectors have been developed, most of them consisting of plastic shields or foam pads, which are kept in place by pockets within specially designed underwear (Figure 1). Several randomized trials have evaluated the effectiveness of hip protectors among patients at risk of hip fractures; however, conflicting results have been reported. At this stage there is no evidence of effectiveness of hip protectors from studies with individual randomization. Data from cluster-randomized studies indicate that, for those living in institutional care with a high background incidence of hip fracture, a programme of providing hip protectors appears to reduce the incidence of fractures. Acceptability of hip protectors by users still remains a problem, mainly due to discomfort and practicality.

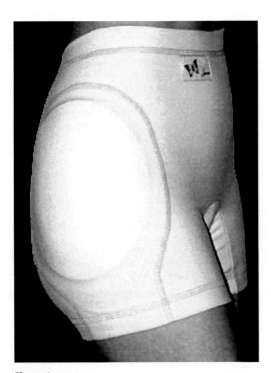

Figure 1
Hip protector. Reprinted with permission from HipSaver Inc., Canton, MA, USA.

Coronary heart disease

Before the menopause, women have a much lower incidence of coronary heart disease (CHD) than men of the same age. With advancing age, the magnitude of sex difference in mortality from CHD decreases. The reasons for the lower incidence of CHD in younger women are not clear. The loss of oestrogen may contribute to the higher risk of heart disease after menopause. Exercise has a direct effect on the cardiovascular system by increasing oxygen delivery and utilization and by decreasing the risk of ventricular arrhythmias and the overall risk of sudden cardiac death. The indirect effects of exercise in modifying risk factors for CHD (for example, decreases in body weight) may be the most important factor in diminishing risk. Exercise therefore may be an effective way to prevent cardiovascular disease in postmenopausal women. The optimal type frequency and intensity are, however, uncertain. A recent study showed that low intensity exercise walking can reduce the risk of cardiovascular disease by about 12–40% over 3.2 years, to a degree similar to that achieved with more vigorous physical activity. This should motivate inactive sedentary postmenopausal women, who may find it easier to undertake walking than more vigorous activities.

Urinary incontinence

Urinary incontinence is another common postmenopausal problem that can be improved by physical exercise. Epidemiological surveys showed that the peak prevalence of stress incontinence occurs around the time of the menopause, and 70% of incontinent postmenopausal women have been reported to relate the onset of their incontinence to the time of their final menstrual period. Physical modalities for stress incontinence are believed to work by strengthening the pelvic floor muscles, so that more pressure can be applied to the urethra, and/or improving coordination of the muscles, so that the urethra has better support when needed (for example, during coughing). A wide variety of physical exercises are used in the treatment of incontinence; these include pelvic floor muscle training (PFMT) and weighted vaginal cones.

Pelvic floor muscle training

Pelvic floor muscle training (or individual voluntary pelvic floor muscle contractions) is the most common form of conservative treatment for stress urinary incontinence. The content of PFMT programmes, however, is highly variable, and the optimal number of exercises needed each day has not been determined. Traditionally, patients have been instructed about pelvic muscle exercises with written or verbal instructions, but, as many women are not able to contract their pelvic floor muscles voluntarily, a thorough assessment of pelvic floor function and training by digital vaginal examination is warranted. Improvement in continence with PFMT is gradual, taking from four weeks to six months. A Cochrane review compared the effects of PFMT on symptoms or urodynamic diagnoses of stress, urge and mixed incontinence with no treatment or other treatment options. Pelvic floor muscle training seemed to be an effective treatment for women with urinary incontinence. Due to limitations of the available evidence it was difficult to judge if PFMT was better or worse than other treatments. Evidence on the effect of adding other adjunctive treatments to PFMT (for example, vaginal cones) equally was limited. The study concluded that further, larger, high-quality trials are needed to determine the real value of physical modalities for the treatment of urinary incontinence. The role of PFMT in the prevention of future continence problems is an area in which more research is needed.

Vaginal cones

The use of weighted vaginal cones is another method to train pelvic floor muscles to improve urinary incontinence. The typical set includes five cones of graduated weights that range from 20 g to 65 g. Starting with the lightest, the woman places the cone in her vagina while standing and tries to prevent the cone from falling out by contracting the pelvic floor muscles. As with PFMT, frequent repetition is needed. Improvement in continence with cones is reported as 60–90%, which is similar to that from other methods, such as PFMT. Poor continuation rates have been reported during treatment, however, which might limit the benefit of these devices to highly self-motivated women.

Further reading

Bonaiuti D, Shea B, Iovine R, et al. Exercise for preventing and treating osteoporosis in postmenopausal women (Cochrane Review). In: *The Cochrane Library, 2003, Issue 4*. Chichester: John Wiley, 2003.

Brownson RC, Eyler AA, King AC, et al. Patterns and correlates of physical activity among US women 40 years and older. *Am J Public Health* 2000; **90**: 264–70.

Coupland CA, Cliffe SJ, Bassey EJ, et al. Habitual physical activity and bone mineral density in postmenopausal women in England. *Int J Epidemiol* 1999; **28**: 241–6.

Cummings SR, Nevitt MC, Browner WS, et al. Risk factors for hip fracture in white women. Study of Osteoporotic Fractures Research Group. *N Engl J Med* 1995; **332**: 767–73.

Feskanich D, Willett W, Colditz G. Walking and leisure-time activity and risk of hip fracture in postmenopausal women. *JAMA* 2002; **288**: 2300–6.

Gregg EW, Pereira MA, Caspersen CJ. Physical activity, falls, and fractures among older adults: a review of the epidemiologic evidence. *J Am Geriatr Soc* 2000; **48**: 883–93.

Hay-Smith EJ, Bo Berghmans LC, Hendriks HJ, et al. Pelvic floor muscle training for urinary incontinence in women (Cochrane Review). In: *The Cochrane Library, 2001, Issue 1*. Chichester: John Wiley, 2001.

Hay-Smith J, Herbison P, Morkved S. Physical therapies for prevention of urinary and faecal incontinence in adults (Cochrane Review). In: *The Cochrane Library, 2002, Issue 2*. Chichester: John Wiley, 2002.

Herbison P, Plevnik S, Mantle J. Weighted vaginal cones for urinary incontinence (Cochrane Review). In: *The Cochrane Library, 2000, Issue 2*. Chichester: John Wiley, 2002.

Kerr D, Morton A, Dick I, Prince R. Exercise effects on bone mass in postmenopausal women are site-specific and load-dependent. *J Bone Miner Res* 1996; **11**: 218–25.

Kohrt WM, Ehsani AA, Birge SJ, Jr. Effects of exercise involving predominantly either joint-reaction or ground-reaction forces on bone mineral density in older women. *J Bone Miner Res* 1997; **12**: 1253–61.

Krall EA, Dawson-Hughes B. Walking is related to bone density and rates of bone loss. *Am J Med* 1994; **96**: 20–6.

Manson JE, Greenland P, LaCroix AZ, *et al*. Walking compared with vigorous exercise for the prevention of cardiovascular events in women. *N Engl J Med* 2002; **347**: 716–25.

McGinnis JM. The public health burden of a sedentary lifestyle. *Med Sci Sports Exerc* 1992; **24**: S196–200.

Moehrer B, Hextall A, Jackson S. Oestrogens for urinary incontinence in women (Cochrane Review). In: *The Cochrane Library, 2003, Issue 4*. Chichester: John Wiley, 2003.

Gormley EA. Biofeedback and behavioral therapy for the management of female urinary incontinence. *Urol Clin North Am* 2002; **29**: 551–7.

Parker M, Gillespie L, Gillespie W. Hip protectors for preventing hip fractures in the elderly (Cochrane Review). In: *The Cochrane Library, 2003; Issue 4*. Chichester: John Wiley, 2003.

Roberts SE, Goldacre MJ. Time trends and demography of mortality after fractured neck of femur in an English population, 1968-98: database study. *BMJ* 2003; **327**: 771–5.

Stevens JA, Powell KE, Smith SM, *et al*. Physical activity, functional limitations, and the risk of fall-related fractures in community-dwelling elderly. *Ann Epidemiol* 1997; **7**: 54–61.

Van Schoor NM, Smit JH, Twisk JW, *et al*. Prevention of hip fractures by external hip protectors: a randomized controlled trial. *JAMA* 2003; **289**: 1957–62.

15 Changing social structures

Leila Hellevi Toiviainen

Introduction

Many changes in social structures today benefit younger and older people because they involve choices that were not available to earlier generations. Retirement ages are more flexible, so individuals can choose to retire earlier and pursue hobbies and engage in a variety of leisure activities or stay in work longer. Many people can extend their careers and remain generally vital later in life because of better living conditions and healthcare than was the case decades ago.

As women work and have gained more independence, they have the choice of not marrying at all or getting divorced more easily than a generation ago. They can exercise more choices in their working and private lives; this results in widened social networks and community involvement. Education is more available through organizations such as the University of Third Age or the Internet.

The less beneficial changes to social structures that affect all members of society are the increasing numbers of older people with lessening resources to meet their needs. Although people live longer and are healthier, a proportion of people in the oldest group of 'people in their eighties and beyond' have multiple physical and cognitive health problems that need complex care.

Members of changing societies need to address the socioeconomic and ethical questions about how they best meet the needs of the most vulnerable individuals in their midst. It is in the interests of the young and the old to have the best possible quality of life, while at the same time, no particular groups or individuals should be disadvantaged. Intergenerational justice should be promoted in the planning and delivery of social policies.

Social changes and individuals

In recent decades in the developed west, the welfare state has taken care of its members by planning and implementing social and health policies that have enhanced the quality of people's lives and have promoted longevity. These measures include the existence of a publicly funded healthcare and pensions provisions. This has been the case in Sweden, which is regarded by many as the paradigm of a western welfare state because of its progressive legislation. Since the 1980s, however, state services for older people have been cut back. As a result, adult daughters especially have to take care of their ageing parents and at the same time, the support services to informal carers also has declined.

In Australia, two thirds of the 2.3 million inhabitants or 10% of the population who are

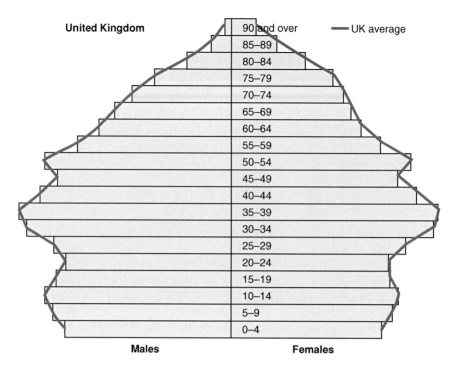

United Kingdom

90 and over
85–89
80–84
75–79
70–74
65–69
60–64
55–59
50–54
45–49
40–44
35–39
30–34
25–29
20–24
15–19
10–14
5–9
0–4

UK average

Males　　　　　　　　**Females**

Figure 1
The age distribution of the UK population in 2001. Adapted from UK census data 2001.

caring for others informally are estimated to be women. Estimates are that this 'invisible workforce' saves the economy $16 billion a year and delivers 74% of services, compared with programs subsidized by federal and state governments for a paltry $1.1 billion a year to meet 9% of the need'.

Caring for parents or relatives

The economic and psychological costs to individual carers of ageing parents or relatives are high. This limits carers' opportunities to take on paid work or adds stress when they try to reconcile the demands of work and caretaking activities. In particular, women who are wives and mothers often have to give up their own employment to care for an older family member. This results not only in loss of income but also in 'lower emotional wellbeing' as a result of being excluded from social contacts through work and interests outside the home. If the parent cared for is confused, the carer has to expend mental and physical effort at the cost of family life.

Similar statistics on the costs of informal caring are available in the UK, where over 5.7 million people care for someone over the age of 75 years (Figure 1). Of these carers, 3.3 million are female and 60% devote at least 20 hours a week to caring. Daughters-in-law report the highest level of stress associated with caring because of past and present relationship problems with their in-laws. Biological daughters of ageing parents, on the other hand, consider themselves natural carers motivated by love for their parents. In many cases, these daughters live with their parent and 'provide more hours of care and are less likely to have a partner or responsibilities to a family of their own'.

Divorce

In contrast with the single women living with and caring for their parents, many older people today experience divorce after 55 years of age. As a result, relationships with their children, as well as with other members of society, change in positive and negative ways. According to a Dutch study, older divorced men are most socially isolated as a result of divorce and retirement. At the same time, many divorced older people in good health find other partners with whom they can share new families and extended social networks. Through these, their lives are enriched. New interests and activities, friends and acquaintances, stepchildren and step-grandchildren add to the newly remarried or 'repartnered' people's sense of wellbeing and belonging. At the same time, these fresh networks may be a source of conflict with the children of new partners: they may bring with them duties towards in laws and thus more of the stresses they escaped from after leaving previous relationships.

Employment

The rapidly changing social structures and diversity of roles demand adaptive skills by the young and the old who need to be more flexible in their private and working lives. No person can rely on having secure, fulltime employment until retirement age. For some, freelance employment in later life provides a viable alternative way to work and live. Mature people with particular expertise and skills can choose self-employment and offer their services to a variety of enterprises rather than working fulltime for one employer: this is known as 'flexible employment' or a 'portfolio career'.

Research conducted into freelance work in the media industry shows that creative professionals can extend their careers by these means. This not only brings them added income but also provides the intellectual challenges that enhance mental and physical wellbeing. For less skilled individuals flexible employment is merely a synonym for financial and job insecurity.

Sexuality

Although western societies have become more permissive in their attitudes to the sexuality of the young, the topic is discussed less often in relation to older people: sex is assumed to no longer play a significant role in their lives. For instance, the Dutch study had no mention of sexuality, even though the issues of companionship and diverse living arrangements are most relevant to repartnering.

A Finnish guide to the good care of older people, however, included a chapter on how health professionals can support the maintenance of the sexual identity of older people. The author emphasizes the fact that older people remain sexual beings, even if the significance and expressions of sexuality change. Older couples may not engage in regular sexual intercourse but rather express their feelings through affectionate acts of caring for their partners. Sexuality at any age cannot be defined merely as sexual intercourse but as a psychic source of strength and an essential feature of self-esteem.

Another Finnish author discussed all of the following as features of the sexuality of older people, although, of course, they should be expressed in intimate relationships at any age:

- love and understanding
- discussion
- knowledge
- imagination
- playfulness and humour

- acceptance
- compassion
- honesty
- reliability.

Sexuality in later life, then, includes the continuing need for physical closeness with a partner and the desire to give and receive affection in all of its forms. It also means having someone with whom to share your concerns. Sexuality is an expression of people's engagement with a vital life force: it enriches the lives of the young and the old.

Conclusion

Changing social structures have brought new freedoms to the young and the old. They can exercise more choices in terms of employment and personal relationships. In some instances, however, changes in attitudes have not kept pace with these changes. Even if older people are able to get divorced and remarry more easily than in past decades, their continuing sexuality is not appreciated as a meaningful part of the new relationships. They should be regarded as agents, not victims, of change in society, through their contribution to public lives of work and contributions to community as wives, husbands, partners and carers, as well as in their private lives lived in increasingly creative and unique ways.

Further reading

National Statistics. *Census 2001*. London: National Statistics, 2001 (http://www.statistics.gov.uk/census2001).

Giervelid J, Peeters A. The interweaving of repartnered older adults' lives with their children and siblings. *Ageing Society* 2003; **23**: 187–205.

Johansson L, Sundstrom G, Hassing B. State provision down, offspring's up: the reverse substitution of old-age care in Sweden. *Ageing Society* 2003; **23**: 269–80.

Legge K. Sensitive old age guys. *Weekend Australian Magazine* 20–21 Sep 2003: 28–32.

Lyonette C, Yardley L. The influence on carer wellbeing of motivations to care for older people and the relationship with the care recipient. *Ageing Society* 2003; **23**: 487–506.

Platman K. The self-designed career in later life: a study of older portfolio workers in the United Kingdom. *Ageing Society* 2003; **23**: 281–302.

Sax S. *Ageing and public policy in Australia*. Sydney: Allen and Unwin, 1993: 31–43.

Schofield H. Family caregivers: disability, illness and ageing. Sydney: Allen and Unwin, 1998.

Suni A. Love and Sexuality. In: Sihvola T, ed. *Grow old wisely: gerontology for the aged*. Saarijarvi: Gummerus, 1995: 49–54.

Voutilainen P, Varama M, Backman K, *et al*. *The good care of ageing individuals: a guide to quality*. Saarijarvi: Gummerus, 2002: 35–6.

16 Counselling and stress management

Dani Singer

Grief that does not speak whispers across the overwrought heart' & bids it break

(Shakespeare)

Introduction

Stress is a complex response to change. Stressors can be subjective and internal – related to perception and expectation – or they can be related to environmental and physiological factors. Stressors may be acute or chronic, current or the result of an accumulation of stressors from childhood, adolescence and early adulthood. Common feature of stress are often associated with the menopause (Box 1).

Box 1
Common symptoms and signs of stress
- Raised blood pressure
- Sleep and gastrointestinal disturbance
- Increased irritability and 'negative' emotions
- Tension, backaches
- Palpitations
- Headaches
- Increased alcohol/caffeine/nicotine use

Menopause as a stressor

The midlife menopause transition can be viewed as a common stressor that is also a normative life event. Sandwiched between youth and old age, this time potentially proffers a greater sense of achievement, fulfillment and understanding and a positive opportunity for revision of the sense of self. It may also be stressful and confusing, without a clearly demarcated roadmap and beset by new and generally unwelcome stressors: biological, psychological and social.

For both genders, midlife is characterized by a shift in responsibility, with similar stressors and symptoms – yet women seem to become more distressed by them. This may be because menopause is linked to sex and reproduction, so that the interpretation and response to bodily changes are influenced by sociocultural issues, as well as personal meaning. The midlife transition may be more problematic in the USA and UK, where physical appearance carries a high social premium, than in Sweden. Recent studies in Sweden showed that most women report increased feelings of freedom and viewed the menopause as a time for development and increased self-esteem. This is also true of several African and Asian cultures, where menopause increases social status and fewer 'negative' symptoms are reported.

Previous studies have linked stress to the secretion of cortisol-releasing hormones during the menopause. Stress and menopause have also been associated with depression, negative mood and memory difficulties, although a direct causal relationship between menopausal symptoms and stress remains unclear.

Measures of stress have ranged from experimental animal studies to the consideration of hidden stressors, such as perception of attractiveness and self-confidence. The latter may be more insidious than those closer to the surface: whether the result of major life changes or the cumulative effects of minor daily irritations, the perception of change (and an adverse reaction to it) are what create a stress response.

Menopausal stressors

For most women, the menopause is not a particularly traumatic life phase; however, 10–20% do seek help for troublesome symptoms – some of which may persist for up to 10 years

Physiologically, hormonal fluctuations, such as hot flushes, night sweats, palpitations, disturbed sleep and mood swings, can be stressful in themselves. Decreased oestrogen can generate dysphoria, which can increase the stress of life events, which further decreases oestrogen levels, and a cycle of neuroendocrine imbalance may develop. Increased headache at menopause has been linked to difficulty in coping with stress, and stress has been implicated in sleep disturbances. Weight gain, although mainly caused by decreases in metabolic rate and activity, may in part result from high cortisol reactivity in response to stress. Prolonged stress may amplify muscle tension or painful sensations or may become somatized, for example in low back pain, particularly in Asian countries where this may be more socially acceptable. Others have linked stress to frequency, duration and troublesomeness of hot flushes, although the evidence is inconsistent.

The impact of bodily changes may be aggravated by life stressors, such as illness, accidents, poor nutrition and sleep disturbance, and by accompanying feelings of redundancy and loss of femininity associated with the end of reproductive capacity. Additional psychological

stressors involve interpersonal relationships, living arrangements (with others or alone), monotony or lack of stimulation at home or at work, or persistent worry: for example, anxiety about making mistakes and working with mainly younger colleagues. This may also be accompanied by frustration at enforced changes and dread of impending loss or bereavement (for example, of parent or partner).

Chronic stressors, such as divorce or separation, and ongoing conflict or isolation within an intimate partnership, have been shown to be associated with changes in hormone levels, as has caring for a parent or spouse with dementia. Stress generated by conflict within marriage and low perceived social support may account for 24% of variation in menopausal symptomatology. Vasomotor symptoms, insomnia, mood swings and irritability are related to higher levels of perceived stress, as are personality traits such as neuroticism or extroversion, but extroversion is positive in that stressful situations are viewed as a challenge. Usually, negative health consequences result from the combination of four factors:

- a stressor (for example, bereavement or conflict)
- a physical reaction (for example, increased blood pressure or a weakened immune system)
- an absence of positive mediators (for example, supportive relationships) to alleviate the above
- perception or experience of stress over a period of time.

Counselling and stress management

The use of non-medical treatments is gaining ground and is increasingly recommended. Treatments often include exercise, diet, meditation, acupuncture, homeopathic and herbal agents, the benefits of which are discussed in Chapters 7, 8, 9, 12, 13 and 14. Several studies link relaxation therapy to a reduction in hot flushes, although this has not always been shown to be statistically significant.

In the UK, a reluctance to accept counselling still exists, yet evidence is accumulating that psychotherapy and counselling can be effective in alleviating psychological distress and other symptoms. The dynamic interaction between external and internal stressors at this time, both psychologically and on a biochemical level, can be addressed through an individually tailored mix of lifestyle and stress management, cognitive behavioural therapy and other counselling approaches.

Counselling

The key systems to consider are:

- family, friendship network and surrounding community
- phase appropriate developmental tasks
- involvement outside of family in the community
- reassessing career involvement
- confrontation with personal mortality.

How well this phase of life is managed depends on individual resources – both material and psychological – but it necessitates an increased reliance on cognitive capacity rather than physical prowess.

Emotional self-management and a sense of personal control alleviate stress. Counselling can act as a positive resource to support and enhance personal coping strategies, but it is not a panacea. Counselling can be a fraught endeavour: high in raised expectations but often low in quick, tangible results. Most of those who opt for counselling are ambivalent about it. Some view counselling as another 'pit stop', with the expectation of having their problems 'fixed' through some kind of psychological prescription, or have already tried this approach but found the benefits only temporary. Some see it as having no use whatsoever ('how can talking help my

problems?'), while others may resent being referred but attend hoping for a magical solution, and still others attend out of a sense of desperation – an admission of weakness or failure. Women who cut themselves off from their feelings may find it hard to engage, particularly in the gap between sessions. This means that the process may remain predominantly intellectual – all too easily kept in a 'compartment' separate from 'real life'. Those with a great deal of distress or anxiety often need time to talk before contemplating change; here, the danger is that meetings become a series of 'off loadings' about events between sessions rather than an opportunity for thinking and development. If and when these hurdles can be overcome and a non-regressive partnership is established, useful understandings and strategies can emerge that have a positive and enduring impact.

Some women who are in relationships have a sense of living alone in a couple without the children to relate through, whereas those not in a relationship may have a painful sense of isolation. In either case, sexual activity – a well known antidote to stress – may have become lackluster, infrequent or non-existent. Deterioration in existing sexual relationships may relate to external stressors such as redundancy, early retirement, moving house, anxiety about children or, less obviously, to internal markers such as anniversaries, weddings and births, which can rekindle memories and regrets, past terminations, lost pregnancies or struggles with fertility. This is likely to be the case particularly if the woman perceives a lack of support from her partner or if there is a history of extramarital affairs. At the same time, aging parents may serve as a reminder of declining health and ultimate loss – a future reflection of the aging body.

Stress management

A problematic menopause experience and its appraisal can also be approached through stress management, incorporating deep breathing and progressive relaxation techniques. Strategies that are misguided (as in social withdrawal) or self-destructive (as in substance abuse) evoke negative social stereotypes that undermine self-esteem and widen the gap between a woman's sense of herself as she is and her aspiration.

Counselling and cognitive behavioural therapy generally involve psychoeducational training aimed at identifying and challenging dysfunctional beliefs to foster a more proactive stance to current stressors. Links can be demonstrated between thoughts, feelings and behaviour by identifying automatic negative thoughts and underlying beliefs, marshalling evidence to question and dispute these and replacing them with more helpful ones, which enhance a sense of wellbeing. This can also be illustrated in a concrete way, using a stress monitor.

After addressing immediate needs for information, for example, that bodily symptoms are self-limiting and do not cause physical damage, additional techniques may be used. These include keeping diary records, learning to slow down and anticipate triggers (for example, for hot flushes) and communicating with significant others. Examination of a woman's expectations of herself and/or others, the degree of effort she puts in to the reward experienced, her locus of control and decision latitude and her social support are also significant in this context. Consideration may need to be given to restructuring priorities, reducing tasks to a manageable size, time management, antiprocrastination techniques, problem solving, assertiveness techniques, maintaining perspective and looking for the positive. Interpersonal skills of active listening, taking the other's perspectives, managing emotions and generalizing these to new situations are also involved. Such a pragmatic and individualized approach has been shown to increase sense of coherence, increase self-confidence and produce a more positive outlook and better adaptation. Where there are

underlying unresolved issues from the past, referral to longer term or more specialized help may be appropriate, although this is often hampered by scarce resources.

Generally, those who benefit the most recognize their own contribution to their difficulties, can isolate issues rather than feeling 'everything's always against me', feel more comfortable with people who are struggling than with those who think they've 'got it made' and are motivated to work towards personal change. For a successful outcome, the individual needs to develop 'emotional hardiness', develop a sense of purpose and be open to change in a way that is achievable in their environment.

Conclusions

A growing consensus that vulnerability to stress contributes to worsening menopausal symptoms suggests that change in social attitude accompanied by psychological intervention may be beneficial. For professionals, this may mean challenging their own and the woman's internalized stereotypes, which pathologize and devalue menopausal women, to enable women to be seen as positive examples of personal growth by themselves, contemporaries and the next generation.

Midlife can be a dynamic phase of life. The potential of counselling and stress management to have an impact, not only on the immediate symptoms of dysfunction but also on longer term capacities suggests that women should have easy access to such support.

Further reading

Berg G, Tottvall T, Hammar M, Lindgreen R. Climacteric symptoms in women aged 60–62 in Linkoping, Sweden. *Maturitas* 1998; **10**: 193–9.

Bertero C. What do women think about menopause? A qualitative study of women's expectations, apprehensions and knowledge about the climacteric period. *Int Nurs Rev* 2003; **50**: 109–18.

Bishop B, Foster A, Klein J, O'Connell V. *Challenges to Practice*. London: Karnack, 2002.

Bosworth HP, Bastian IA, Rimer BK, Siegler IC. Coping styles and personality domains related to menopausal distress. *Women's Health Issues* 2003; **13**: 32–8.

Busch H, Barth-Olofsson AS, Rosenhagen S, Collins A. Menopausal transition and psychological development. *Menopause* 2003; **10**: 179–87.

Calvaresi E, Bryan J. Symptom experience in Australian men and women in midlife. *Maturitas* 2003; **44**: 225–36.

Chilvers C, Dewey M, Fielding K, *et al*. Antidepressant drugs and generic counselling for treatment of major depression in primary care: randomised trial with patient preference arms. *BMJ* 2001; **322**: 772.

Dennerstein L, Iehert P, Burger H, Dudley F. Mood and the menopausal transition. *J Nerv Ment Dis* 1999; **187**: 685–91.

Epel E, Lapidus R, McEwen B, Brownell K. Stress may add bite to appetite in women: a laboratory study of stress-induced cortisol and eating. *Psychoneuroendocrinology* 2001; **26**: 37–49.

Griffin M. The sexual health of women after the menopause. *Sexual and Marital Therapy* 1995; **10(3)**: 277–91.

Hodson J, Thompson J, Al-Azzawi F. Headache at menopause and in hormone replacement therapy users. *Climacteric* 2000; **3**: 119–24.

Hunter M. Cognitive behavioural interventions for premenstrual and menopausal symptoms. *J Reprod Infant Psychol* 2003; **21**: 183–93.

Jones CR, Czajkowski L. Evaluation and management of insomnia in menopause. *Clin Obstet Gynecol* 2000; **43**: 187–97.

Kuh DL, Wadsworth M, Hardy R. Women's health in midlife: the influence of the menopause, social factors and health in earlier life. *Br J Obstet Gynaecol* 1997; **104**: 923–33.

Mazure CM, Bruce ML, Maciejewski PK, Jacobs SC. Adverse life events and cognitive personality characteristics in the prediction of major depression & antidepressant response. *Am J Psychiat* 2000; **57**: 896–903.

North Carolina Department of Medicine. Coping styles and personality domains related to menopausal stress. *Women's Health Issues* 2003; **13**: 32–8.

Powell LH, Lovallo WR, Matthews KA, *et al*. Physiologic markers of chronic stress in premenopausal middle-aged women. *Psychosomat Med* 2002; **64**: 502–9.

Reynolds F. Exploring self-image during hot flushes using a semantic differential scale: associations between poor self-image, depression, flush frequency and flush distress. *Maturitas* 2002; **42**: 201–7.

Schneider HP. The quality of life in the post-menopausal woman. *Best Pract Res Clin Obstet Gynaecol* 2002; **16**: 395–409.

Seligman ME, Schulman P, DeRubeis RJ, Hollon SD. The prevention of depression and anxiety. *Prevention & Treatment* 1999; **Vol 2**: Article 8.

Taechakraichana N, Jaismrarn U, Panykhamlerd K, *et al*. Climacteric concept, consequence and care. *J Med Assos Thailand* 2002; **85 (suppl 1)**: 1–15.

Wijma K, Melin A, Nedstrand F, Hammar M. Treatment of menopausal symptoms with applied relaxation: a pilot study. *J Behav Exp Psychiatry* 1997; **28**: 251–61.

Woods NF, Mitchell ES. Pathways to depressed mood for midlife women: observations from the Seattle Midlife Women's Health Study. *Res Nurs Health* 1997; **20**: 119–29.

Woods NE, Mitchell ES, Adams C. Memory functioning among midlife women: observations from the Seattle Midlife Women's Health Study. *Menopause* 2000; **74**: 257–65.

Yip Y, Ho SC, Chan S. Socio-psychological stressors as risk factors for low back pain in Chinese middle-aged women. *J Adv Nurs* 2001; **36**: 409–16.

Index

Page numbers in *italics* refer to information in figures or tables

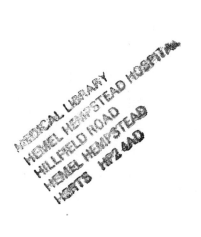